KT-215-060

# THE HAIRY DIETERS

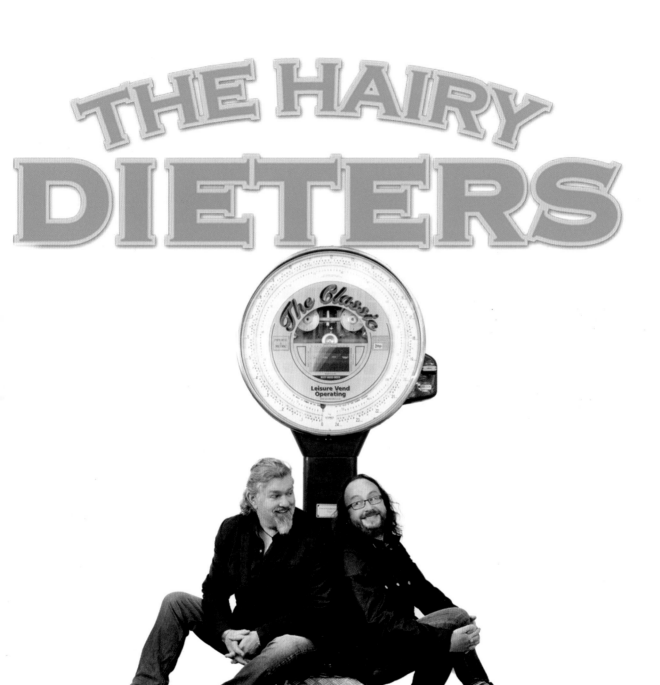

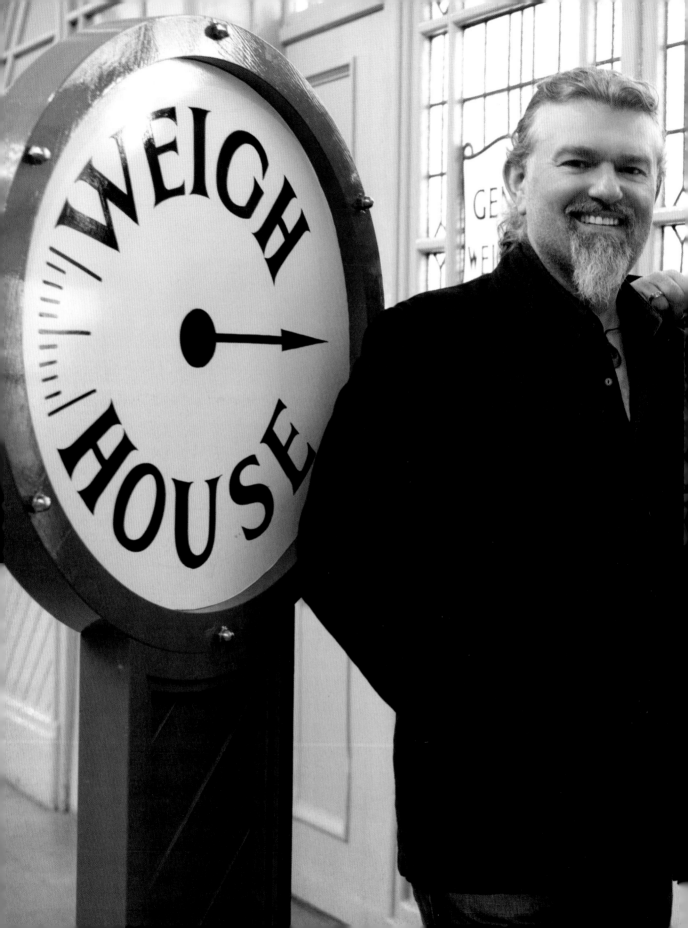

Si King & Dave Myers

# THE HAIRY
# DIETERS

WEIDENFELD & NICOLSON

We'd like to dedicate this book to our families and friends, who've put up with our grumpiness and newfound sobriety. If we do say so ourselves, we are looking the better for it, though. Short-term pain for long-term gain.

First published in paperback in Great Britain in 2012 by
Weidenfeld & Nicolson, an imprint of the Orion Publishing Group Ltd
Orion House, 5 Upper St Martin's Lane, London WC2H 9EA
an Hachette UK Company

40 39 38 37 36 35 34 33 32 31

Text copyright © Byte Brook Limited and Sharp Letter Limited 2012
Design and layout copyright © Weidenfeld & Nicolson 2012
The Hairy Dieters programme, programme material and format copyright © Optomen Television Ltd, 2012

All rights reserved. Apart from any use permitted under UK copyright law, this publication may only be reproduced, stored or transmitted, in any form, or by any means, with prior permission in writing of the publishers or, in the case of reprographic production, in accordance with the terms of licences issued by the Copyright Licensing Agency.

A CIP catalogue record for this book is available from the British Library.

ISBN: 978 0 297 86905 4

Photographer: Andrew Hayes-Watkins
Food stylist: Lisa Harrison, with Anna Burges-Lumsden
Prop stylist: Giuliana Casarotti
Designer: Loulou Clark
Food and recipe consultant: Justine Pattison
Editor: Jinny Johnson
Proofreader: Elise See Tai
Indexer: Elizabeth Wiggans
Photographer's assistants: Zoe Russell, Kristy Noble
**Nutritional analysis calculated by:**
Fiona Hunter (BSE Hons Nutrition Dip Diet) and
Lauren Brignell ( BSC Hons Nutrition)

**Optomen Television production team:**
Executive producer: Nicola Moody
Series producer and director: Ian Denyer
Food consultant: Justine Pattison
Home economist: Jane Gwillim

Printed in Italy by Printer Trento

Every effort has been made to ensure that the information in the book is accurate. The information in this book will be relevant to the majority of people but may not be applicable in each individual case so it is advised that professional medical advice is obtained for specific health matters. Neither the publisher and authors or Optomen accept any legal responsibility for any personal injury or other damage or loss arising from the use or misuse of the information in this book. Anyone making a change in their diet should consult their GP especially if pregnant, infirm, elderly or under 16.

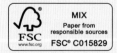

optomen

BBC logo is a trademark of the British Broadcasting Corporation and is used under licence. BBC logo © BBC 1996.

# CONTENTS

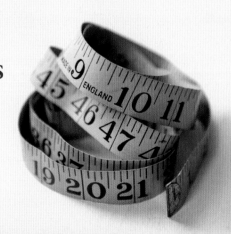

Food isn't just fuel for us – it's our life. We spend most of every day cooking, thinking about food and coming up with recipe ideas, not to mention eating! Great-tasting food is our passion and we're not about to give that up.

But we have to admit that we've overdone it a bit. Years of enjoying endless gorgeous meals has taken its toll and we've piled on the pounds. Like many middle-aged blokes – and ladies – we found that we'd got too hefty and our health was suffering. It was time to face facts and take a good hard look at ourselves so we took a deep breath and got on the scales. Ouch! It was a long time since we'd weighed anything except ingredients and it was a shock. We were both a couple of stone or more overweight and over 40% of our body mass was fat. It was time to diet.

Now we have to be honest, we're never going to be skinny minnies and we don't want to be. It's just not us. But we've made the effort to lose weight to stay healthy and enjoy life to the full. We want to be walking up hills and down dales without getting out of breath, and to be riding our big bikes when we're 70 so we need to keep mobile and trim. And that means every now and again watching what we eat and reining it in a bit.

Okay, we're not going to diet for ever – we're still greedy and we'll always love our pies and curries – but our weigh-in was a wake-up call to act before we got dangerously big. Losing weight has been quite a journey for us but we've done it and we're proud of ourselves. Now we know we can drop the pounds when we need to and this will help us keep a check on things in the future. If we can do it so can you.

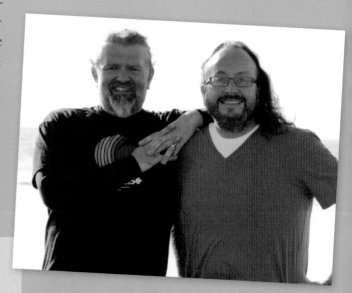

*Look at losing weight as an investment in yourself and the people you love. The benefits far outweigh the sacrifices.*

**Si:** *"I was always chubby, even as a lad. I ate for comfort after my dad died when I was only eight years old and the weight just continued to pile on. I didn't know when to stop. I got teased at school, but I kept on eating. At 11 years old I was 11 stone. By my 12th birthday I was 12 stone. And then when I got into this game, I had every excuse to eat the most fantastic food whenever I wanted."*

**Dave:** *" I was quite skinny as a kid, but my mam and dad and me all loved our food. But my dad had a physically demanding job in a paper mill and he burned it all off. My life has been very different, but I've gone on eating the pies and hot pots and big roasts, as well as the fine dining all around the world. When you're on the road a lot like we are, it's hard to eat sensibly and all too easy to stoke up on rich fatty food. I'm never going to be skinny again but I don't want to be obese either."*

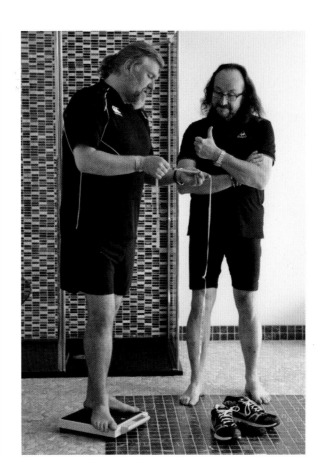

## SO THIS IS WHAT WE DID

We didn't want to sacrifice the pleasure of cooking and feel deprived or hungry so we knew we had to come up with meals that we would enjoy making and eating if we were to stick with the diet.

With the advice of healthy eating experts, we discovered that by making small changes in our cooking habits we could still enjoy big flavours and the food we loved while dropping the pounds. And it's true. We've shed weight and we feel the better for it. Our blood pressure and cholesterol levels are down, our waistlines have shrunk, we have more energy and we look HOT – but not as sweaty as we used to!

And even more importantly, we've done all this while still eating some of our favourite, great-tasting dishes that we now cook with less fat and sugar, but bags of flavour.

We think our recipes are fantastic. Yes, they're lower in fat and sugar but they still taste amazing and we're still just as enthusiastic and creative about our cooking as ever.

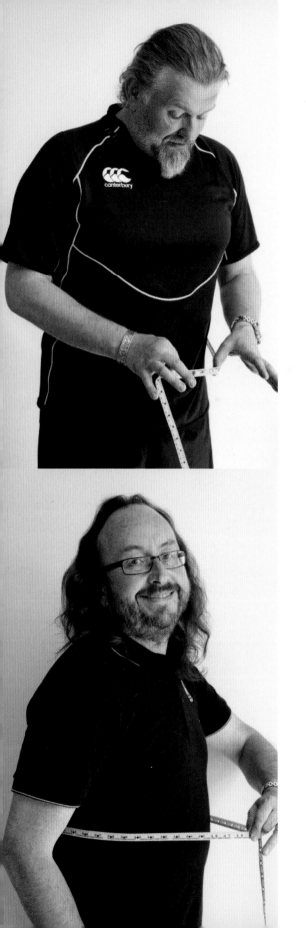

# COUNTING THE CALORIES – IT'S WORKED FOR US AND IT CAN WORK FOR YOU

We've found a way of eating ourselves slimmer and we want to share our discoveries with you. The secret is to make better choices and use little tricks to reduce your daily calorie count. Calorie counting might have fallen out of favour somewhat over recent years, replaced by all sorts of wacky dieting ideas, but it does work. We're the living proof. We've lost pounds and inches!

We've made all the recipes in this book as low in calories as possible while not compromising on the taste. And we've had a nutritionist check them out and do calorie counts for each one so you know exactly where you are. If you eat these, without cheating, you will lose weight – and you'll love us for it.

We have to confess we've never really thought too much about calories and the amount of food we were taking in but we know a lot more now. As many as a quarter of us Brits are obese and it's not good for us, so it seems that many of us are taking in much more than we're putting out.

**Our experts explained to us that in order to lose weight, you have to take in fewer calories so the body has to use its stores – makes sense so far doesn't it?**

The average man needs about 2,500 calories a day and the average woman about 2,000. That does, of course, vary according to how active you are, your build and other factors. For instance, if you work on a building site, you use more calories than if you're sitting at an office desk.

We were told that to lose a kilo (about 2 pounds) a week we should cut our calorie intake by at least half – to 1300–1500 calories a day – and that's what we've done. Before we started the diet, we kept a food diary for a few days and the results were quite something. We realised that we were scoffing about 3,500 a day before and that was way, way too much.

## LOSE WEIGHT WITH US

Cook the recipes in this book, don't cheat on portion size or extra snacks and you will lose weight too. But we're not experts – we just know what's worked for us – so we recommend that you check with your doctor before starting any diet. When you reach your target, relax a little – but not too much – and continue to weigh yourself once a week. The minute the scales start to creep up, get a bit stricter with yourself and get back on track.

**Once you've achieved your weight loss, treat this book as your maintenance manual, your everyday cook book, to help you keep in shape.**

## CALORIES

A calorie is a unit of energy contained in food – you'll see the calorie count listed on lots of types of packaged food. We burn calories to produce energy, but if we take in more than we need, they're stored as fat.

On packages you'll see calories given as kilocalories, the proper name, but don't worry, they're the same thing. On some packages you will also see a figure in kilojoules, another way of measuring food energy. This will be a larger figure (there are over 4 kj in one calorie) so don't be alarmed. Calories are all you need to worry about for the recipes in this book.

Bear in mind that calorie counts on packaged food are usually for a serving, not for the whole pack, and one brand can vary from another.

# OUR TIPS FOR A SKINNIER YOU

- Buy some good scales and weigh yourself once a week. Weigh yourself first thing in the morning, after you've had a wee. We've found we can weigh as much as kilo more in the evening.

- Once you've reached your target weight, keep checking regularly and go back on the plan if you find you've gained a few pounds. It's a whole lot easier to lose two pounds than two stone.

- Buy a full-length mirror, if you don't already have one. Get your kit off, stand in front of it and take a good long look at yourself.

- Rethink your eating habits with the help of the recipes in this book. You can still enjoy lots of your old favourites if you cook them in a slightly different way to make them lower in calories but with full-on flavour.

- Reduce the amount of fat you eat – and that means oil as well as butter. There are 9 calories in a gram of fat, whatever kind it is.

- Exercise might not take off the pounds by itself, but does make you feel healthier, fitter and more energetic.

- Make carbs the smallest portion on your plate. Choose wholegrains and cut right down on starchy white carbs, such as white bread, pasta, rice and potatoes. If you're making a sandwich, go topless – use one slice of bread instead of two. When you make mash, mix in some leeks or cabbage to make it go further.

- Spice things up. Spicy food is full of flavour so we reckon it helps you feel more satisfied. No need for diet food to be bland or boring – the chilli is the dieter's friend.

- Eat protein. It fills you up and keeps you going. Don't forget, though, that cheese is fat.

- Be sure to eat breakfast, have a good lunch and a meal in the evening. Make this a habit.

- If you give way to temptation one day and overdo it, don't despair and give up. Just be extra strict with yourself the next day to make up for it. It's like your bank balance – if you slip into the red, it's payback time. Think of your meal plan over a week, rather than day by day.

# THE DEMON DRINK

It's dead hard, we know, but it's important to avoid alcohol if you want to encourage and maintain your weight loss. All types of alcoholic drinks are full of empty calories – and if you do give in and have a couple of drinks you're more likely to throw caution to the winds and guzzle down more food.

Instead, drink mainly water; fizzy or still. Add a dash of angostura bitters to your fizzy water when you want a bit of a change if you like. And if you want the occasional low-calorie fizzy drink, such as diet cola, that's fine too, but limit your diet drinks to just a couple a day or you may find any sweet craving you have could worsen. Look on it as a bit of a sabbatical – time out until you've got things under control.

## A FEW POINTERS FROM US

We've given a calorie count per portion for each recipe and we mean per portion. So if the recipe is for two, don't think you can eat the whole lot and have the same calorie count.

Weigh all the ingredients carefully and use proper tablespoons, teaspoons and a measuring jug. This is particularly important for these recipes because if you use more of an ingredient than indicated in the recipe, you'll change the calorie count.

You'll notice that there are quite small amounts of high-cal ingredients, such as Parmesan cheese. That's because the flavour is strong and you don't need a lot. Trust us and don't cheat.

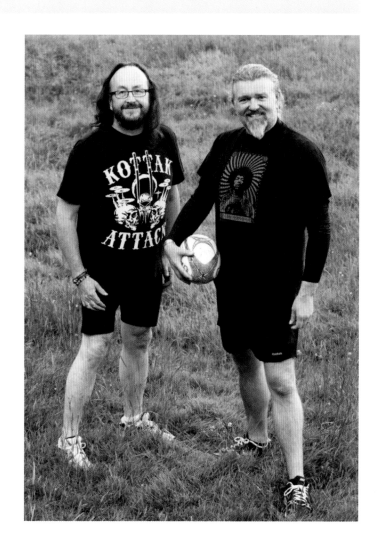

# SI AND DAVE'S WEIGHT-LOSS TIPS

————

Don't skip breakfast. If you don't have time to eat before you leave home, take something with you to work. Try our home-made muesli or granola with some semi-skimmed milk or low-fat yoghurt.

————

Find something you like and can prepare easily so you don't have too many decisions to make in the morning. We've found that uncertainty can lead to temptation.

————

Other breakfast ideas: a bowl of porridge, made with water or semi-skimmed milk, is good, especially when topped with poached fruit. Another favourite of ours is half a can of baked beans with a couple of slices of ham – it's hot and filling with lots of fibre and protein.

————

Making your own granola and muesli puts you in control – you know exactly what's in there.

————

Fresh fruit juice is high in calories so always dilute juice with water.

————

Eggs are a great breakfast and keep you feeling full for longer. Try boiled or scrambled egg with a slice of wholemeal toast. You can have egg and bacon, but poach the egg, leave out the toast and hash browns and fill up with mushrooms and grilled tomatoes instead. A slice of ham makes a nice change from bacon.

————

# BREAKFAST & BRUNCH

"The cold hard truth is that the only way to lose weight is to eat less of the bad stuff and more of the good."

*Dave*

# TOASTED CRUMPETS AND WARM
# SPICED BERRIES WITH YOGHURT AND HONEY

*You'd think crumpets were a big no-no when dieting, but it's not the crumpets that are the problem – it's the butter you usually slather on to them. Top your crumpets with this mixture of gooey fruit, honey and yoghurt and you'll never miss the butter.*

**SERVES 2**

4 crumpets
100g fat-free Greek yoghurt
150g ripe strawberries,
hulled and sliced
50g raspberries
50g blueberries
2 big pinches of ground mixed spice
2 tsp runny honey, for drizzling

*257 calories per portion*

Toast the crumpets in a toaster or under the grill until lightly browned. You don't want a flabby crumpet, so make sure you toast them well. Put the yoghurt in a bowl and stir until it looks glossy.

Place a non-stick frying pan over a medium-high heat and add all the fruit. Sprinkle with 2 good pinches of ground mixed spice and cook for just a minute, tossing regularly until the fruit is softened but still holding its shape. This will bring out the sweetness without the need to add extra sugar.

Divide the hot, toasted crumpets between 2 plates. Spoon the fruit over the top and allow some of it to tumble on to the plates. Spoon the yoghurt on top and drizzle with a little honey. Eat right away.

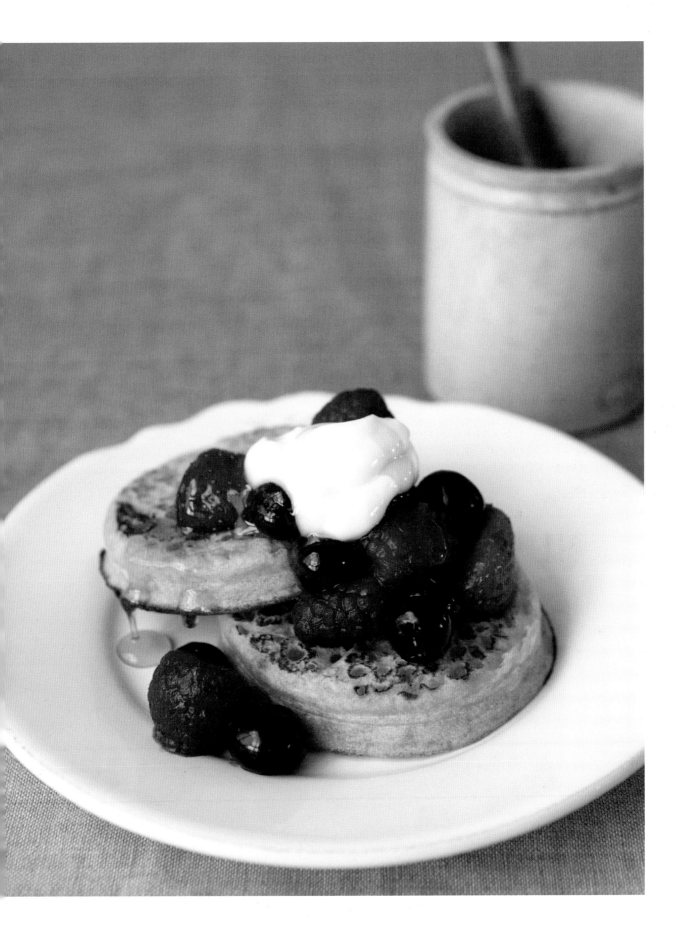

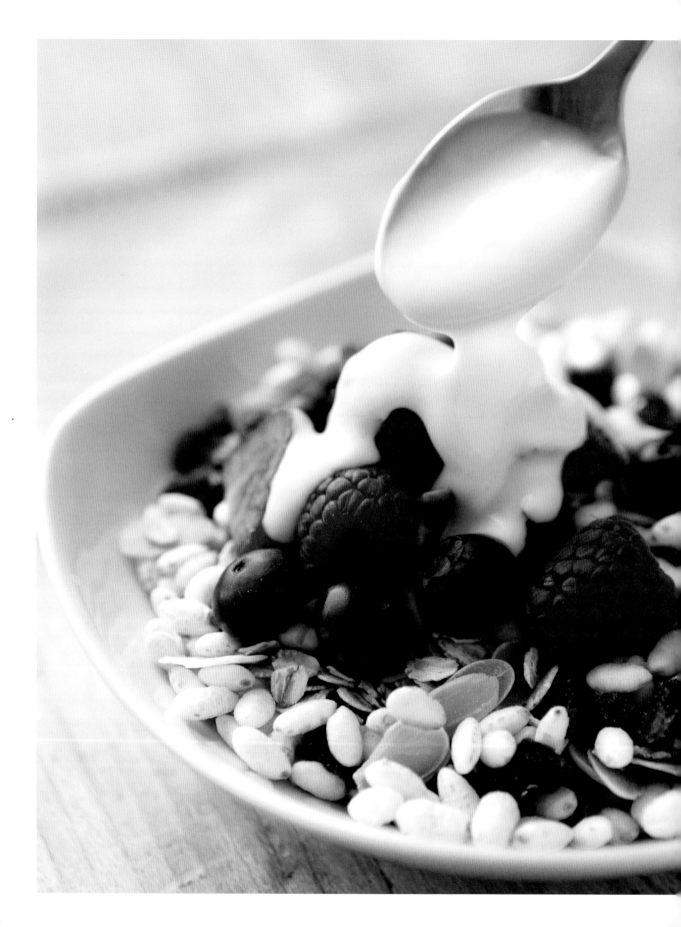

# CRANBERRY AND ALMOND MUESLI

*Making your own muesli is easy and you know exactly what's in it – loads of good stuff and no rubbish. We find this mixture makes a smashing breakfast and, with a handful of fresh fruit and a good dollop of yoghurt, it really keeps you going until lunchtime.*

Place a large non-stick frying pan over a medium heat, add the almonds and toast them for 3–5 minutes, turning occasionally. Keep a careful eye on them so they don't burn. Tip the nuts into a large mixing bowl and allow them to cool slightly.

Pour the oats and puffed rice into a large rubber-sealed jar or plastic food container. Add the toasted almonds, mixed dried fruit and cranberries or sour cherries and mix everything together well.

Enjoy a 50g portion of the muesli for breakfast with semi-skimmed milk or low-fat natural yoghurt and some fresh berries if you like.

**MAKES 12 SERVINGS**

50g flaked almonds
300g jumbo porridge oats
75g unsweetened puffed rice
100g mixed dried fruit
100g dried cranberries or
sour cherries
semi-skimmed milk or low-fat
natural yoghurt, to serve
assorted fresh berries (optional)

*195 calories per portion (without milk)*
*241 calories per portion (with 100ml semi-skimmed milk)*

**Top tip:** *If you do buy muesli, check the packets carefully. We've noticed that some of the luxury products are very high in sugar so watch out. They're not as healthy as they look.*

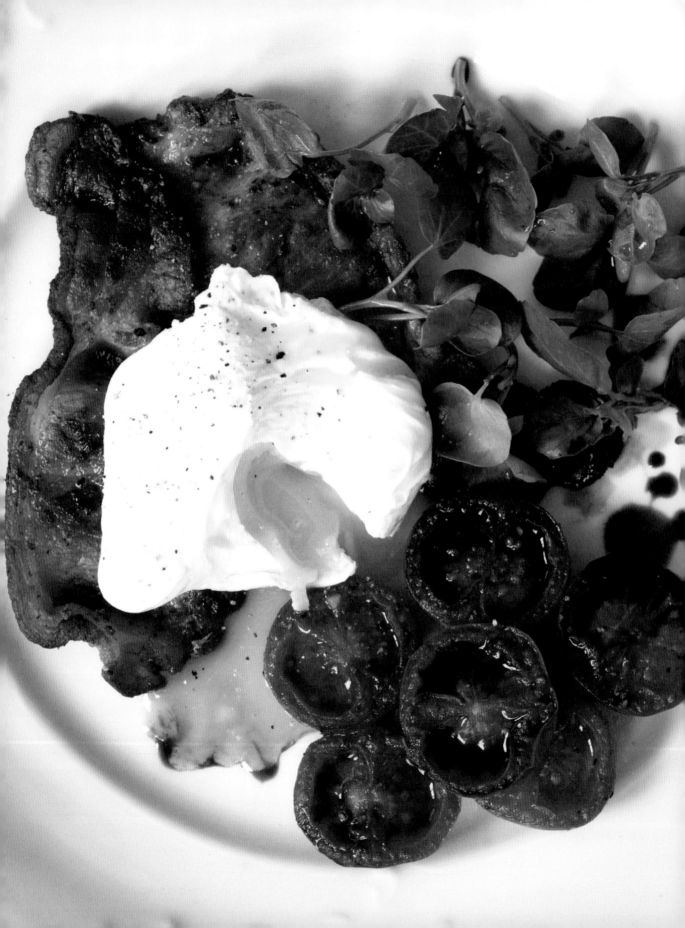

# PAN-FRIED BACON WITH
# POACHED EGG AND BALSAMIC TOMATOES

*Guess what? You don't have to give up your bacon and eggs when you're dieting – just slightly change the way you cook them. Poaching the eggs and dry-frying the bacon saves on fat and the whole dish tastes just as good. Choose good lean bacon and avoid streaky.*

Brush a large non-stick frying pan with sunflower oil, using the tip of a pastry brush. Place the pan over a medium heat and add the bacon. Cook for 2 minutes until lightly browned, then turn and dry-fry on the other side for another 3 minutes.

While the bacon is cooking, half fill a medium non-stick saucepan with water, add the vinegar and bring to the boil. Turn the heat to low, so the water is only just bubbling.

Crack the eggs into the water, 1 at a time, spacing them well apart. Cook for 2½ minutes. The eggs should rise to the surface within a minute. If the egg white sticks to the bottom of the pan, lift it gently with a wooden spoon. Alternatively, you can use a hob-top egg poacher, lightly greased with sunflower oil.

Add the tomatoes to the pan with the bacon and season with plenty of black pepper. Cook the tomatoes for about a minute until just beginning to soften, turning them once. Put a small pile of watercress on each plate.

Place some bacon and tomatoes on the plates and drizzle with a dash of balsamic vinegar. Take the eggs out of the water with a slotted spoon and place them on top. Season with a little more pepper and tuck in right away while it's all lovely and hot.

**SERVES 2**

1 tsp sunflower oil
4 rashers of rindless smoked back bacon
1 tsp white wine vinegar
2 large very fresh eggs (fridge cold)
8 cherry tomatoes, halved
good handful of watercress
drizzle of good-quality balsamic vinegar
freshly ground black pepper

*264 calories per portion*

# SCRAMBLED EGGS
# WITH SMOKED SALMON

*This is a treat – light but tasty and packed with protein. It takes next to no time to prepare and makes a really special weekend breakfast or brunch. Shows that you can breakfast like a king and still keep the calories under control.*

**SERVES 2**

4 medium eggs
1 tbsp freshly snipped chives, plus a few extra to garnish (optional)
15g butter
4 slices of smoked salmon (about 75g)
1 English muffin, cut in half
flaked sea salt
freshly ground black pepper

*354 calories per portion*

Beat the eggs with a pinch of flaked sea salt and lots of freshly ground black pepper. Use a metal whisk and make sure you beat the eggs really well. Stir in the chives if you're using them.

Melt the butter in a medium non-stick saucepan over a low heat. Pour the beaten eggs into the pan and cook very gently for 2 minutes, stirring slowly until the eggs are softly scrambled. Remove from the heat and stir for a few seconds more – the eggs will continue to cook for a while.

While the eggs are cooking, toast the muffin and put 1 half on each plate, cut side up. Spoon the scrambled eggs over the muffins, add the slices of smoked salmon and season with a little more black pepper. Garnish with extra chives if you wish. Serve immediately.

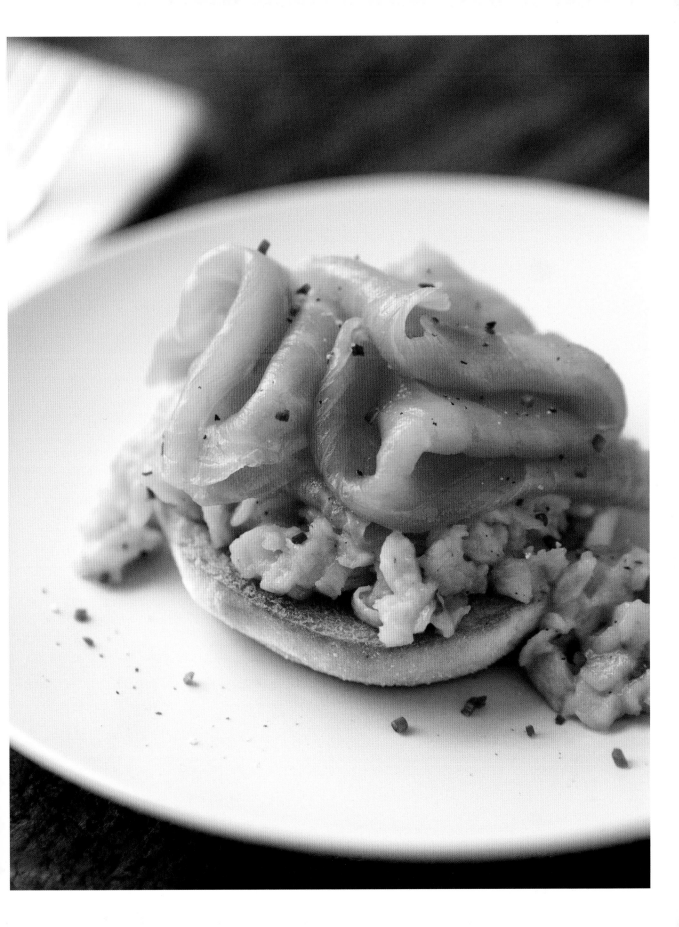

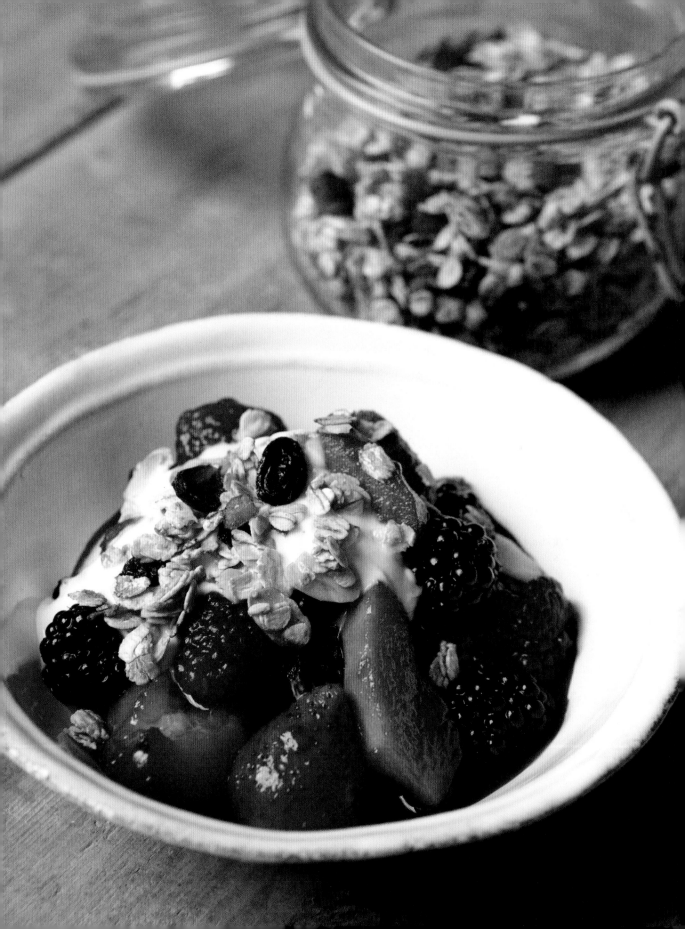

# FRESH FRUIT COMPOTE
# WITH HOME-MADE GRANOLA

*We find a bowl of this compote, topped with some of our special crunchy granola and a spoonful of low-fat yoghurt, sets us up a treat in the morning. It's like sunshine for your insides.*

To make the granola, preheat the oven to 180°C/Fan 160°C/Gas 4. Line a large baking tray with baking parchment.

Pour the apple juice into a medium saucepan and bring to the boil. Continue boiling until the liquid has reduced by two-thirds and is syrupy. It's really important to get this bit right, as the apple syrup needs to be thick enough to lightly coat the oats.

Add the oats and almonds to the pan with the apple syrup and stir until well combined. Tip everything on to the baking tray and spread out thinly. Bake in the centre of the oven for 15 minutes.

Take the tray out of the oven and scatter the dried fruit over the top. Turn and mix everything with a spatula or spoon and put the tray back in the oven for another 5 minutes or until the oats are crisp and lightly golden. Remove from the oven and leave to cool on the tray, then tip the granola into an airtight tin or jar. This mixture is best eaten within 2 weeks.

To make the compote, preheat the oven to 190°C/Fan 170°C/Gas 5. Peel the apples and cut them into quarters. Remove the cores and slice the apples thinly. Put the apples with the plums and half the sugar in a shallow ovenproof dish – a lasagne dish is ideal. Cover loosely with a sheet of foil and bake for 30 minutes.

Take the dish out of the oven and add the whole berry fruits to the dish. Sprinkle with the remaining sugar and toss lightly together. Cover with foil and return to the oven for a further 15 minutes or until the fruit is soft and juicy but still holding its shape – it will continue to cook once you've taken it out of the oven. Leave the compote to cool, then tip it into a bowl and cover with cling film. It will keep in the fridge for up to 3 days.

Serve the compote in bowls, topped with a couple of spoonfuls of the granola and some low-fat yoghurt if you like.

**SERVES 6**

**Home-made granola**
300ml apple juice (we prefer the cloudy type)
150g jumbo porridge oats
15g flaked almonds
50g mixed dried fruit

**Fruit compote**
2 Bramley cooking apples (about 150g each)
4 fresh ripe plums, stoned and cut into quarters
75g golden caster sugar
200g strawberries, hulled
200g raspberries
200g blackberries
6 tbsp low-fat natural yoghurt (optional)

*243 calories per portion (without yoghurt)*
*252 calories per portion (with yoghurt)*

# BAKED HADDOCK, SPINACH AND EGG POTS

*Full of protein and really tasty, this is a luxurious weekend breakfast or brunch dish. We eat it with thin crispbreads, which only have about 20 calories per piece, so you can have a couple for dipping into the egg. Thinly sliced pumpernickel bread is also delicious but will add extra calories to the dish, so go easy.*

**SERVES 4**

200g young spinach leaves
1 tbsp cold water
150g skinless smoked haddock, cut into 2cm cubes
125g half-fat crème fraiche
4 spring onions, trimmed and sliced
2 tsp cornflour
sunflower oil, for greasing foil
4 medium eggs (fridge cold)
grated nutmeg, for sprinkling (optional)
freshly ground black pepper
very thin rye crispbreads, to serve (optional)

*187 calories per portion*

Preheat the oven to 220°C/Fan 200°C/Gas 7. Place 4 x 200ml ramekins on a baking tray. Put the spinach in a large saucepan with the tablespoon of cold water and cook over a medium heat until the leaves are wilted, stirring often. This will take 2–3 minutes.

Tip the spinach into a sieve and press it well with a ladle or the back of a wooden spoon to squeeze out as much water as possible. Transfer it to a bowl and add the haddock, crème fraiche, spring onions, cornflour and lots of freshly ground black pepper. Mix well and divide the mixture between the ramekin dishes.

Cover each dish with lightly oiled foil and bake for 15 minutes until bubbling. Take the dishes out of the oven and stir each one well. Make a dip in the centre of each haddock mixture with the back of a spoon. Break an egg into each ramekin and season with a little ground nutmeg if you like.

Cover with the greased foil once more and put the ramekins back in the oven for about 8 minutes or until the eggs are almost cooked. The egg white should no longer look transparent, but the yolk should be runny. Take the dishes out of the oven, leave the foil in place and allow to stand for a further 2 minutes or until the eggs are almost set. Serve hot with crispbreads.

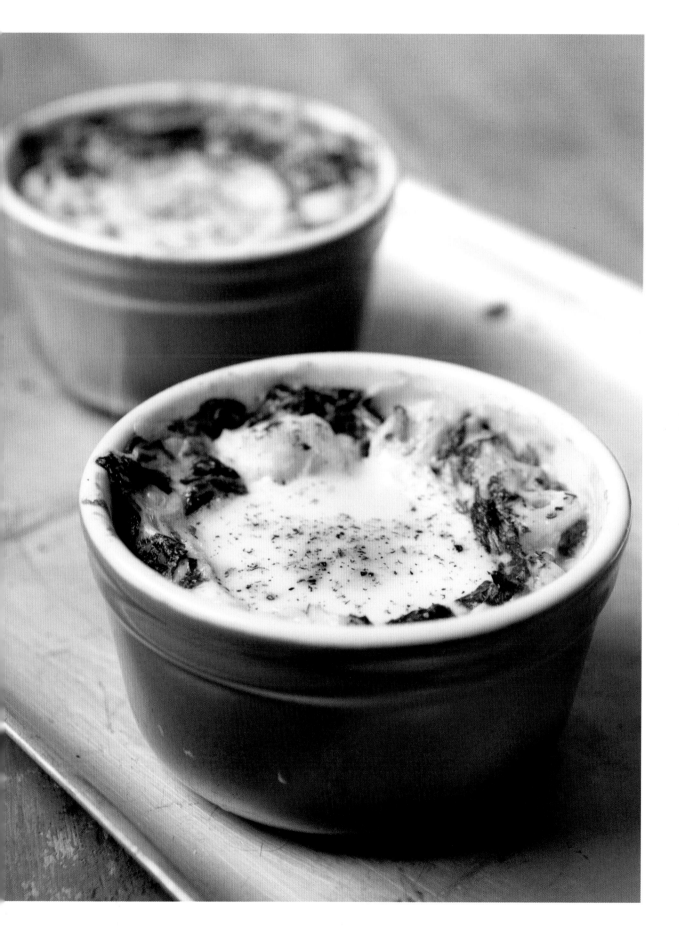

# SI AND DAVE'S WEIGHT-LOSS TIPS

---

Non-stick means less fat. Invest in a really good non-stick frying pan for cooking fish, chicken and other dishes perfectly with the minimum of fat.

---

The recipes in this chapter are all complete meals with a good balance of protein and vegetables and not much carbohydrate.

---

Make your own soup rather than buying it so you are in control of the ingredients. A bowl of soup is comforting, warming and nourishing – a perfect lunch with a hunk of wholegrain bread.

---

Broth-style soups are particularly low in calories but high in taste and you can add loads of green veg – also low in calories.

---

An omelette is the perfect quick meal. Can be filled with anything you have to hand.

---

Peppers, courgettes and tomatoes are great in one-pan dishes and have fewer calories than starchy vegetables such as carrots. They create their own juices as they cook so you don't need to use lots of oil – just a light coating if at all. Using less oil allows you to appreciate the flavour of the food.

---

# ONE-PAN DISHES

"Cook with less fat. You really can get away with using far less butter and oil than you think."

*Si*

# PRAWN AND CHIVE OMELETTE

*Omelettes are a weight-watcher's best friend. If you come in from work ravenous and you're tempted to head for the bread and cheese, knock up an omelette and you'll be sitting down to a fab meal in minutes. Oozing with prawns and chives, this version couldn't be tastier.*

**SERVES 1**

3 medium eggs
1 tbsp freshly snipped chives
100g peeled North Atlantic prawns, thawed if frozen
½ tsp sunflower oil, for brushing
flaked sea salt
freshly ground black pepper

339 calories

Break the eggs into a bowl and beat them with a large metal whisk. Season with a little salt and some freshly ground black pepper, then stir in the snipped chives. Drain the prawns in a sieve, then tip them on to some kitchen paper to soak up any excess moisture.

Brush a small non-stick frying pan with just enough oil to lightly coat the base and place it over a medium heat. Pour the eggs into the frying pan. As the eggs begin to set, use a wooden spoon to draw the cooked egg towards the centre. Do this 5 or 6 times, working your way around the pan. As the cooked egg is moved, the uncooked egg will run into the gaps and begin to cook.

Scatter the prawns over the omelette and cook for a further 2–3 minutes or until the eggs are just set. Season with a little more pepper, then carefully loosen the sides with a heatproof palette knife and fold the omelette over. Slide it on to a warmed plate and serve with a large, lightly dressed salad.

*Top tip:* Instead of prawns, you could add some thinly sliced ham or fresh tomato quarters and a handful of spinach.

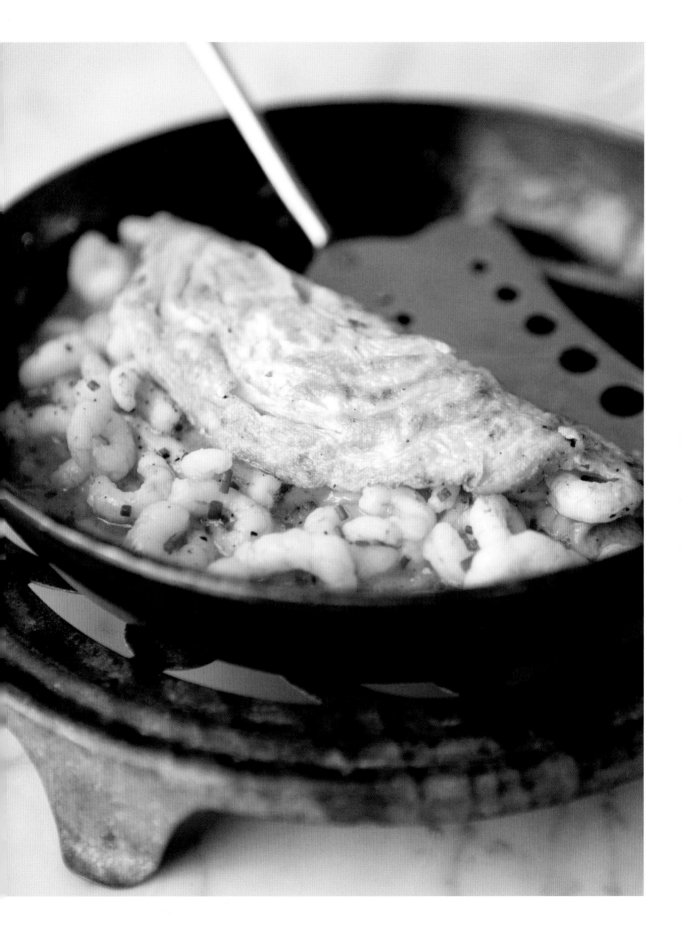

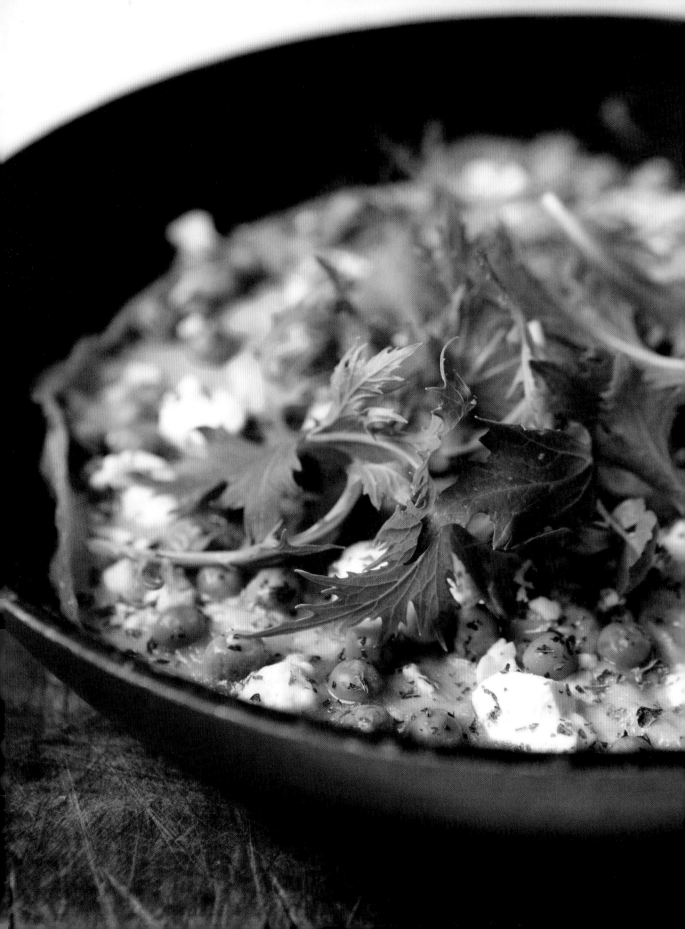

# MINTED PEA AND FETA OMELETTE

*Normally you need to be careful about adding cheese to an omelette as it can really pile on the calories. Feta has such strong taste, however, that you can get away with adding very little and still get the benefit of the fab flavour.*

Put the peas in a heatproof bowl and pour over enough just-boiled water to cover. Leave for a minute, then drain the peas in a sieve and tip them back into the bowl. Crumble the feta cheese on top, sprinkle over the mint and season with lots of freshly ground black pepper.

Break the eggs into another bowl and beat them with a large metal whisk. Season with a little salt and some freshly ground black pepper. Brush a small non-stick frying pan with just enough oil to lightly coat the base and place it over a medium heat.

Pour the eggs into the frying pan. As the eggs begin to set, use a wooden spoon to draw the cooked egg towards the centre. Do this 5 or 6 times, working your way around the pan. As the cooked egg is moved, the uncooked egg will run into the gaps and begin to cook.

Scatter the peas and feta over the omelette and cook for another 3 minutes or until the eggs are just set. Carefully loosen the sides with a heatproof palette knife and slide the omelette on to a warmed plate, folding it as you do so. Serve with a large, lightly dressed salad.

**SERVES 1**

30g frozen peas
40g feta cheese, drained
½ tsp dried mint
3 medium eggs
½ tsp sunflower oil, for brushing
flaked sea salt
freshly ground black pepper

---

382 calories

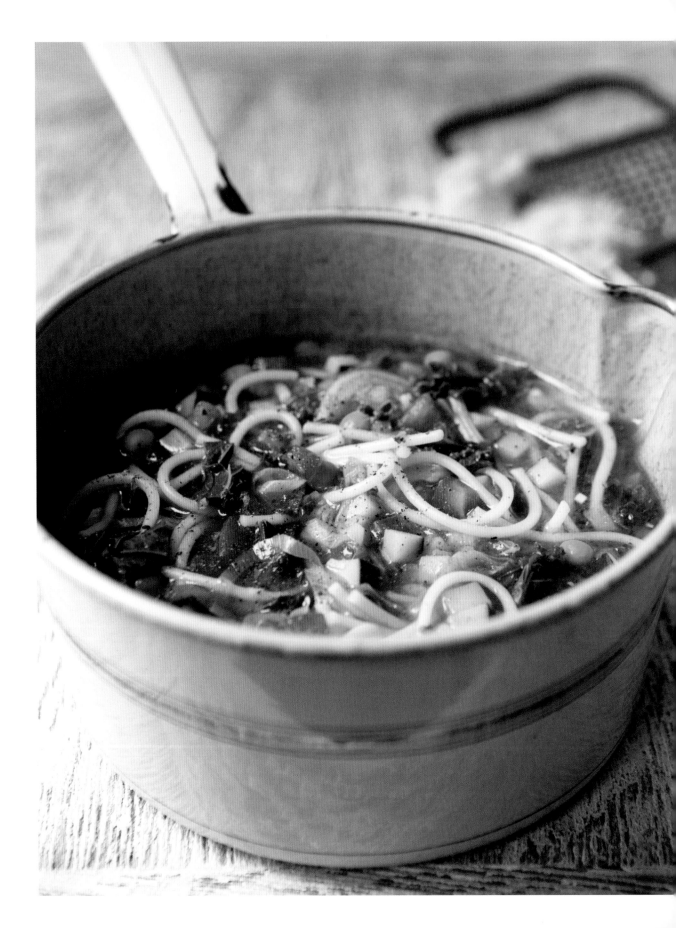

# MINESTRONE SOUP

*A steaming bowl of this makes a super-satisfying lunch with a slice of crusty wholemeal bread on the side. Low in fat but high in flavour, soup is also a good staple to keep in the fridge. Pop a mugful in the microwave when your cravings get too much for you.*

Make a cross in the bottom of each tomato and put them in a heatproof bowl. Pour over enough just-boiled water to cover the tomatoes and leave for 1 minute. If the tomatoes are ripe enough, the skins should shrink back under the hot water. Drain and leave to cool.

Heat the oil in a large non-stick saucepan or sauté pan and fry the onion very gently for 5 minutes until softened but not coloured, stirring often. While the onion is cooking, slip the skins off the tomatoes and cut the flesh into quarters. Scoop out the seeds and chuck them out. Cut the tomato flesh into rough 1cm cubes.

Add the celery, garlic, leek and courgettes to the pan with the onion. Stir over a low heat for a couple of minutes, then stir in the chopped tomatoes, pour over the chicken stock and bring to the boil.

Break the spaghetti into short lengths and drop them into the pan. Add the tomato purée and bring the soup back to the boil, then cook for 8 minutes, stirring occasionally. Add the peas, kale or cabbage and cook for another 5 minutes or until the pasta is just tender.

Season the soup with salt and lots of freshly ground black pepper. Serve with a sprinkling of Parmesan and torn basil leaves if you like.

**SERVES 6**

4 ripe tomatoes
2 tsp olive oil
1 small onion, finely chopped
1 celery stick, finely sliced
2 garlic cloves, peeled and finely sliced
1 slender leek, trimmed and finely sliced
2 medium courgettes, diced
1.5 litres chicken stock, fresh or made with 1 chicken stock cube
50g dried spaghetti
1 tbsp tomato purée
200g frozen peas
100g curly kale or green cabbage, thickly shredded
25g Parmesan cheese, finely grated (optional)
fresh basil leaves, to garnish (optional)
flaked sea salt
freshly ground black pepper

*98 calories per portion*
*115 calories per portion (with Parmesan)*

# GOLDEN VEGETABLE SOUP

*There's nothing like a bowl of home-made soup on a cold day – it feels properly comforting and sustaining. This hearty soup has a great velvety texture which we both love. Just the thing to chase away your dieting blues.*

**SERVES 6**

1 small butternut squash (about 850g)
4 medium carrots (about 375g)
2 medium parsnips (about 325g)
1 medium onion
2 garlic cloves
2 tsp sunflower oil
1 litre just-boiled water
1 vegetable or chicken stock cube
freshly ground black pepper
low-fat natural yoghurt and freshly snipped chives, to serve (optional)

*102 calories per portion*

Peel the squash, cut it in half, then scoop out the seeds. Chuck the seeds away and cut the squash flesh into rough 3cm chunks. Peel the carrots and parsnips and cut them into 2cm slices. Peel and roughly chop the onion and the garlic.

Heat the oil in a large non-stick saucepan and gently fry the onion and garlic for 10 minutes until softened and lightly coloured, stirring occasionally. Stir in the squash, carrots and parsnips. Pour over the just-boiled water, crumble the stock cube on top and bring to the boil. Turn down the heat slightly and simmer the vegetables for 25–30 minutes or until they are completely tender, stirring occasionally.

Remove the saucepan from the heat and blitz the soup with a stick blender until smooth – or leave it a little chunky if you prefer. Alternatively, let the soup cool for a few minutes and blend it in a food processor, then tip it back into the pan. Warm the soup through, then ladle it into warmed bowls. Season with some black pepper and top with a swirl of yoghurt and a few snipped chives if you want to make it look a bit more fancy.

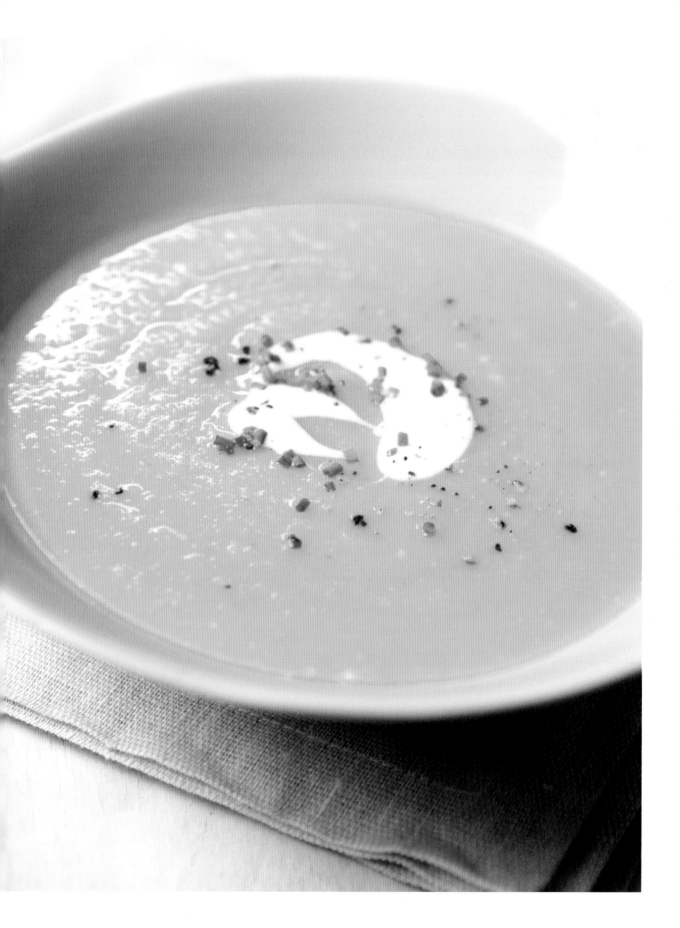

# MUSHROOM, FETA AND TOMATO BAKED PEPPERS

*It's always important for food to look good, whether you're dieting or not, and these peppers are a delight to the eye as well as the tastebuds. A great vegetarian recipe, this has lots of strong flavours that come together in a beautifully colouful and well-balanced dish.*

**SERVES 2**

4 sun-dried tomato pieces in oil, drained well
2 tsp sunflower oil
175g chestnut mushrooms, wiped and diced
20g blanched hazelnuts, roughly chopped
1 garlic clove, peeled and crushed
50g dry white breadcrumbs
½ small bunch of parsley, leaves finely chopped
1 tsp dried chilli flakes
100g feta or soft goat's cheese, drained
2 smallish peppers, red or yellow
freshly ground black pepper

*401 calories per portion*

Preheat the oven to 220°C/Fan 200°C/Gas 7. Roughly chop the sun-dried tomatoes. Heat the oil in a large frying pan and stir-fry the mushrooms over a high heat for 4 minutes.

Add the roughly chopped hazelnuts and fry for a further minute until the nuts are lightly toasted. Season with a good grind of black pepper and remove from the heat.

Stir in the tomatoes, garlic, breadcrumbs, parsley and chilli flakes until thoroughly combined. Break the cheese into small chunks and toss them through the stuffing lightly. Cut the peppers in half from top to bottom and carefully remove the seeds and membrane.

Place the peppers in a small foil-lined roasting tin, cut side up, and fill each half with the mushroom and feta stuffing. Cover the surface of the stuffing with a small piece of foil. Bake for 35 minutes until tender, removing the foil for the last 10 minutes of the cooking time. Serve warm with a lightly dressed mixed salad.

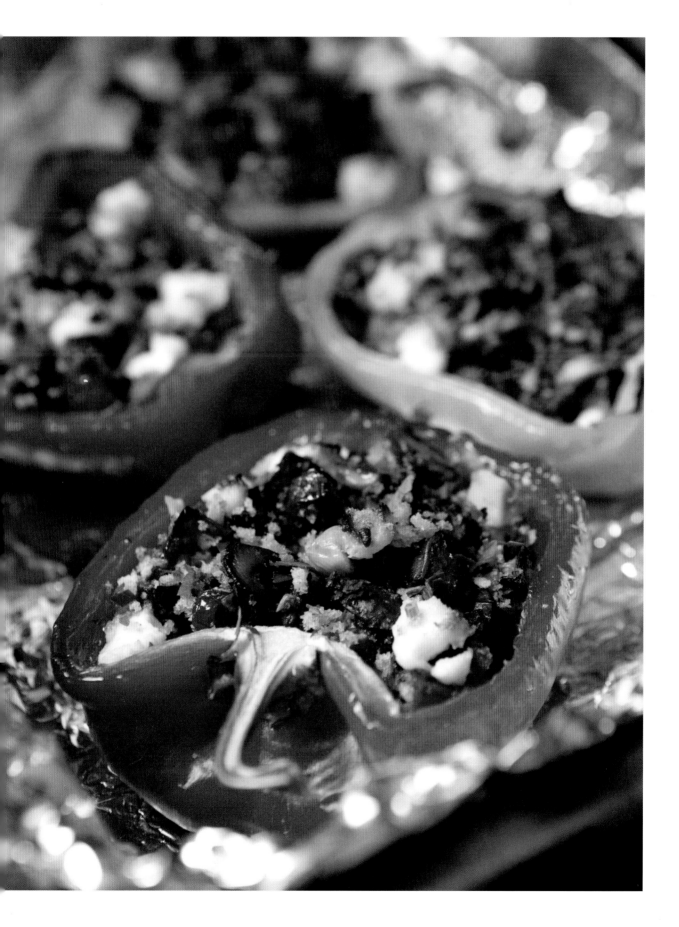

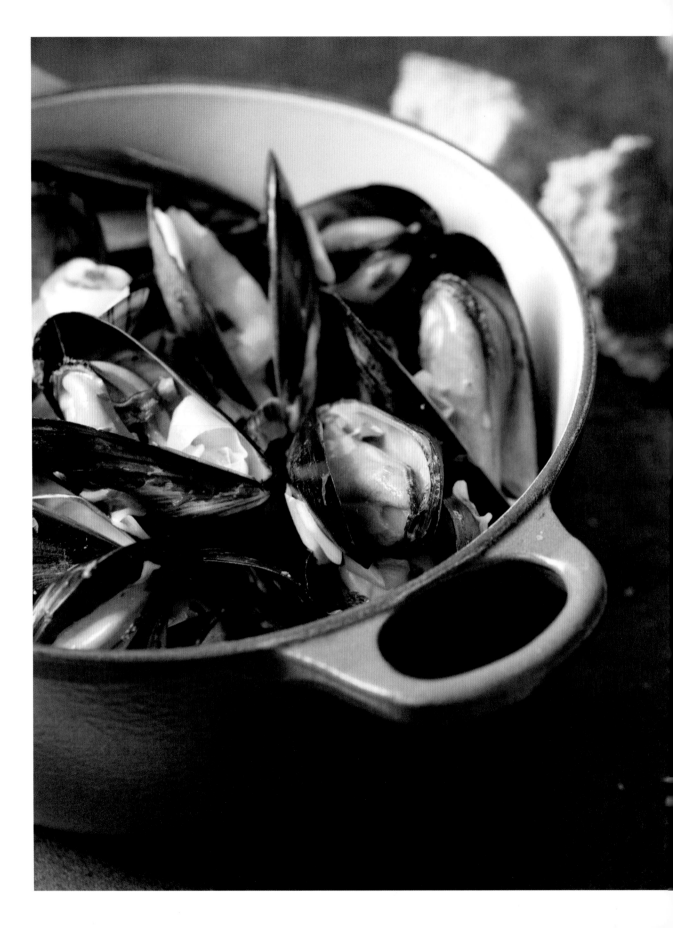

# MUSSELS WITH LEEKS AND WHITE WINE

*Mussels are a favourite of ours. They're a great dish when you're trying to lose a bit of weight, as they are low in calories but high in taste. They take a while to eat too, so help you feel satisfied. And as we all know, the ladies like a man with more muscles than fat!*

Scrub the mussels really well and remove their stringy beards. Chuck out any mussels that are damaged in any way or that are open and don't close when tapped on the side of the sink.

Heat the oil in a large non-stick frying pan or sauté pan – you need something with a lid – over a low heat. Very gently fry the leeks and garlic for 5 minutes until softened but not coloured, stirring occasionally. There's no need to cover the pan. Add a little water to the pan if the leeks start to stick before they are softened.

Pour over the white wine and stir in the crème fraiche and parsley. Add the mussels, cover the pan with a lid and cook for 3–4 minutes or until all the mussels have steamed open, stirring once. Give the pan a good shake now and again. Mix the cornflour and water together to make a thin paste.

Remove the pan from the heat and tip the mussels and their liquor into a colander over a large bowl. Throw away any that haven't opened, then divide the mussels between 2 warmed wide bowls.

Tip the mussel liquor back into the pan and stir in the cornflour paste. Bring to a simmer and cook for 1 minute, stirring until thickened. Add a bit more salt and pepper to taste and pour the sauce back over the mussels in the bowls.

Serve each bowl of mussels with a thick slice of crusty bread for mopping up the sauce. Heaven!

### SERVES 2–3

1kg fresh live mussels
2 tsp sunflower oil
2 slender leeks, trimmed and cut into 1cm diagonal slices
2 garlic cloves, peeled and finely sliced
150ml white wine
4 tbsp half-fat crème fraiche
small handful of flat-leaf parsley, leaves roughly chopped
1 tsp cornflour
1 tbsp cold water
2 thick slices of crusty wholegrain bread
flaked sea salt
freshly ground black pepper

*387 calories per portion (if serving 2)*
*252 calories per portion (if serving 3)*

*Top tip:* *The cornflour paste makes the sauce thicker and creamier which we like, but you can leave it out if you prefer.*

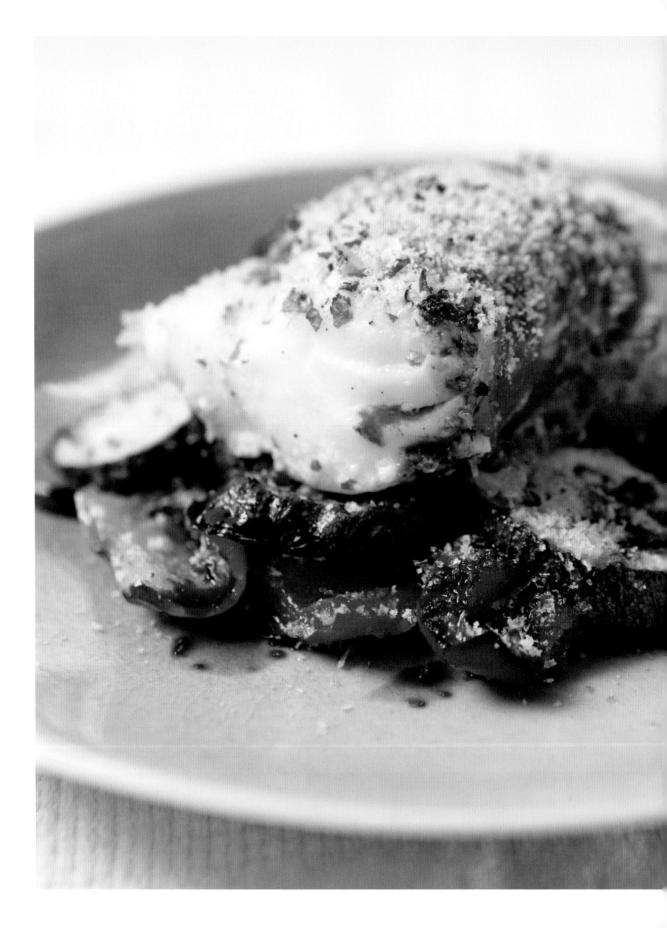

# ROASTED COD WITH PARMA HAM AND PEPPERS

*Cod works really well for this recipe, as it has nice firm flesh, but you can use any white fish. Make sure the fillets are all about the same size so they cook evenly. This couldn't be easier to prepare but tastes really special. It's so good you won't miss the chips.*

Preheat the oven to 220°C/Fan 200°C/Gas 7. Put the peppers, courgettes and onion in a large baking tray and drizzle them with the oil. Season with a little salt and plenty of ground black pepper and toss everything together until the vegetables are lightly coated with oil. Roast for 20 minutes until softened and lightly charred.

Pat the fish dry on kitchen paper and check for any bones. Remove any that you see with tweezers. Season the fish with freshly ground black pepper and wrap each fillet loosely with a slice of ham.

Take the baking tray out of the oven and make gaps in the layer of vegetables to make space for the pieces of fish. Place the fish on the tray. Mix the breadcrumbs with the cheese and parsley and scatter over the fish and vegetables.

Put the tray back in the oven for another 12–15 minutes or until the fish is cooked, the ham has crisped and the breadcrumbs are lightly browned. Serve hot, drizzled with a little balsamic vinegar.

**SERVES 4**

1 red pepper, deseeded and cut into 3cm chunks
1 yellow pepper, deseeded and cut into 3cm chunks
2 medium courgettes, trimmed and cut into 2cm slices
1 medium red onion, cut into thin wedges
1 tsp olive oil
4 x 150g thick skinless cod (or other white fish) fillets
4 slices of Parma ham or any thinly sliced prosciutto
10g dry white breadcrumbs
10g Parmesan cheese, finely grated
2 tbsp finely chopped parsley
2–3 tsp good quality balsamic vinegar
flaked sea salt
freshly ground black pepper

*224 calories per portion*

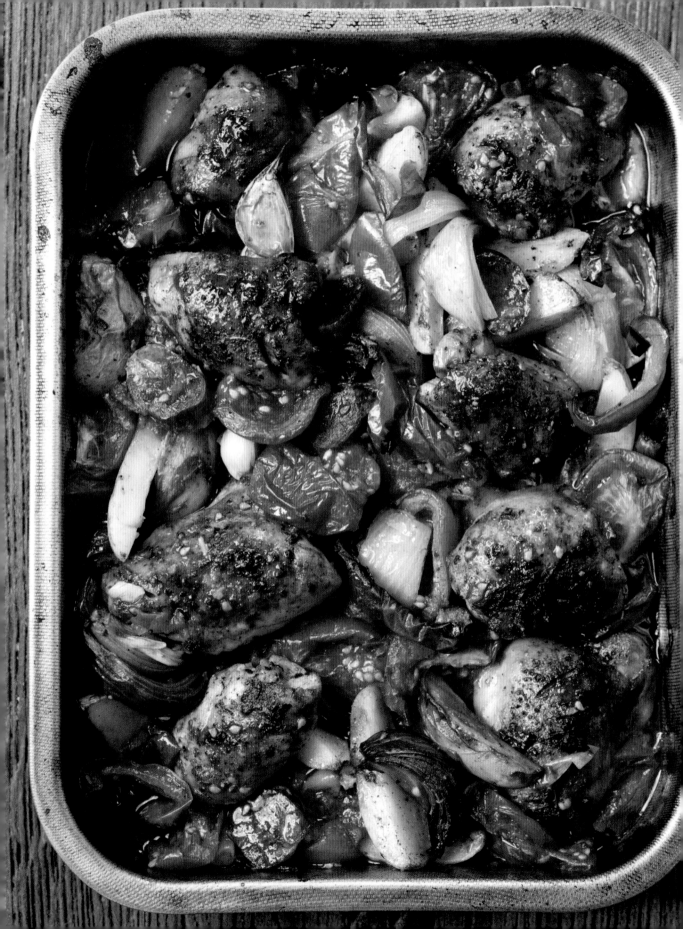

# SPANISH-STYLE CHICKEN BAKE

*This is a brilliant recipe and you'll notice that there's no additional fat needed – all the fat comes from the chorizo, and the tomatoes make it lovely and juicy. A low-fat fiesta of a dish.*

Preheat the oven to 200°C/Fan 180°C/Gas 6. Put the onions, potatoes, garlic and tomatoes in a large roasting tin and season with sea salt and lots of freshly ground black pepper. Toss everything together lightly and roast for 20 minutes.

While the vegetables are roasting, skin the chorizo and cut the meat into thin slices – 5mm is about right. Put the chicken thighs on a board and carefully slash each one 2 or 3 times with a knife. Season all over with black pepper. Mix the paprika and oregano together and set aside.

Take the roasting tin out of the oven, scatter the chorizo over the veg and turn everything a couple of times. Place the chicken on top of the vegetables and chorizo and sprinkle with the paprika and oregano. Season with a little salt and return to the oven for 20 minutes.

Take the tin out of the oven. Holding one corner carefully with an oven cloth, lift the tin a little so all the juices run to the opposite end, then spoon and drizzle the juices back over the chicken. Tuck the pepper strips loosely around the chicken and vegetables.

Turn the oven up to 220°C/Fan 200°C/Gas 7. Put the tin back in the oven for another 20 minutes or until the peppers are just softened and the chicken is golden and crisp. As you eat, squeeze the garlic out of the skins and enjoy the deliciously soft and fragrant flesh. Just don't kiss anyone afterwards!

**SERVES 4**

1 medium onion, cut into 8 wedges
1 medium red onion,
cut into 8 wedges
500g new potatoes,
quartered lengthways
8 whole garlic cloves, unpeeled
8 medium tomatoes, quartered
75g chorizo (preferably picante)
8 boneless, skinless chicken thighs
½ tsp sweet smoked paprika
½ tsp dried oregano
1 green pepper, deseeded and
cut into strips
flaked sea salt
freshly ground black pepper

*370 calories per portion*

# WHOLE BAKED FISH WITH SUN-DRIED TOMATOES

*Don't get fatter, leave off the batter! Baking fish such as sea bass whole is the very best way of cooking them, as it preserves all the flavour and delicious juices. This is a great dish for sharing – put the fish and vegetables on a large platter, take it to the table and dig in. Ask your fishmonger to gut and scale the fish for you. A 675g fish will probably weigh about 550g once prepared.*

**SERVES 2**

1 medium red onion, sliced
1 yellow or orange pepper, deseeded and cut into 3cm pieces
175g new potatoes, cut into 1cm slices
2 tsp olive oil
1 slice of ciabatta bread (about 25g), cut into 1cm chunks
3 sun-dried tomato pieces in oil, drained well
2 garlic cloves, peeled
15g pine nuts (preferably Italian)
handful of fresh flat-leaf parsley, roughly chopped
handful of fresh basil, roughly shredded
1 whole sea bass, gutted and scaled (about 550g once prepared)
freshly squeezed juice of 1 lemon
flaked sea salt
freshly ground black pepper

*417 calories per portion*

Preheat the oven to 220°C/Fan 200°C/Gas 7. Put the sliced onion, pepper and new potatoes on a large baking tray and drizzle with 1 teaspoon of the oil. Season with a little salt and lots of freshly ground black pepper. Toss the veg together well and spread them out on the tray. Bake in the oven for 20 minutes or until the vegetables are lightly browned and beginning to soften.

While the vegetables are cooking, make the stuffing for the fish. Put the ciabatta pieces in a large non-stick frying pan and place it over a medium heat. Cook for 4–5 minutes, turning regularly until the chunks of bread are lightly toasted.

Cut the sun-dried tomatoes into thin strips and finely slice the garlic. Add the pine nuts, garlic and tomatoes to the frying pan and toss together over a low heat for 2 minutes more until the nuts are lightly toasted. Remove the pan from the heat and leave to cool for a few minutes. Add the parsley and basil leaves and toss together.

Working carefully as some sea bass fins are very spiky, slash the fish diagonally with a knife 4 times down each side. Sprinkle with half the lemon juice, making sure plenty goes into each cut and season with black pepper. Take the tray with the vegetables out of the oven and turn them with a spatula. Push the veg into a heap down the centre of the tin and place the fish on top.

Open the fish and spoon the bread, tomato and herb filling inside. Don't worry if a few pieces fall on to the tray but try to keep them close to the fish or they could burn. And remember that the baking tray will be hot, so watch your fingers. Close the fish and drizzle with the remaining lemon juice and the rest of the oil.

Bake for 20–25 minutes or until the fish is just cooked and the filling is hot. Check by sliding a knife into the thickest part of the fish and peering inside – the fish should look white and a little flaky rather than translucent. Serve right away – nothing else needed.

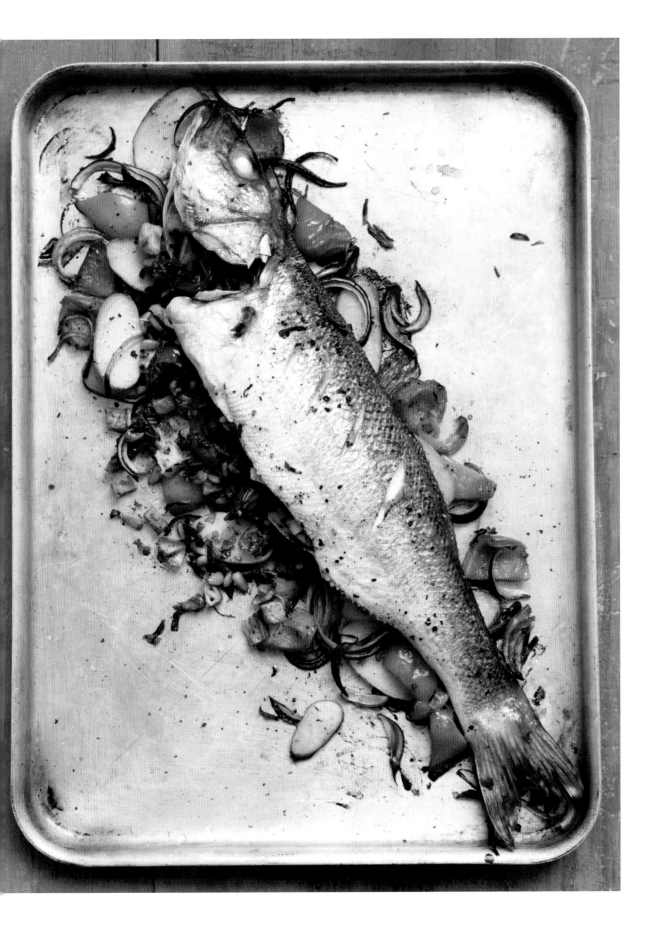

# SI AND DAVE'S WEIGHT-LOSS TIPS

————————

Fine to cook your meat with skin but don't eat it. Much of the fat –
containing lots of calories – lies under the skin.

————————

Roasting can be done with very little fat. Put the meat on a rack so
fat drips off and you can throw it away.

————————

We are not big fans of aerosol spray oils, but if you're lucky enough
to find pure mild olive oil or virgin olive oil in a spritz-style
container, go ahead and use it. Saves brushing the pan with oil.
We've tried filling our own spritz-style oil containers but the nozzles
always seem to get clogged after a couple of squirts.

————————

Bulk out your meals with vegetables so you don't overdo the meat
portions. In our beefburger recipe we add some veg to the mixture
so the meat goes further.

————————

Gammon with parsley sauce is one of our favourites. If you thicken
the sauce with cornflour instead of butter and flour it dramatically
reduces the calorie count but the sauce still tastes good.

————————

Buy yourself a griddle pan. It cooks meat well and the result looks
as good as it tastes. The fat runs into the channels on the pan and
can be chucked out. Barbecuing is great too.

————————

# GRILLS & ROASTS

"Protein is good. It really fills you up and keeps you going."

*Dave*

# SALMON WITH CHILLI GINGER SAUCE

*Oily fish, such as salmon, is a great choice when you're watching your weight, but bear in mind that it contains more calories than white fish. It's a high-quality protein, so fills you up, and it is delicious – especially when teamed with this sticky, tangy sauce. You need to allow time for the fish to marinate for 30 minutes but once that is done, this is quick and easy to prepare.*

**SERVES 4**

2 balls of stem ginger in syrup (and 2 tablespoons of the syrup)

3 garlic cloves

3 tbsp dark soy sauce

finely grated zest of ½ well-scrubbed orange

freshly squeezed juice of 1 orange (about 125ml)

½ long red chilli, thinly sliced

4 x 125–150g salmon fillets, skin on

freshly ground black pepper

*254 calories per portion*

Put the ginger balls on a board and slice them thinly. Pile up the slices from each ball and cut through them to make thin matchstick strips. Put these in a bowl that's large enough to hold the salmon and add 2 tablespoons of the stem ginger syrup from the jar. Peel the garlic cloves and slice them thinly, then add them to the bowl with the ginger. Stir in the soy sauce, orange zest, orange juice and red chilli.

Put the salmon in the bowl with the marinade. Season with lots of ground black pepper and turn a couple of times, ending with the fish skin side up. Cover and chill for 30 minutes.

Preheat the oven to 220°C/Fan 200°C/Gas 7. Line a small baking tray with baking parchment. Take the salmon fillets out of the marinade, scraping off any bits and pieces, and place them on the tray, skin side down. Season with more ground black pepper. Bake for 12–15 minutes, depending on the thickness of the salmon.

While the salmon is cooking, prepare the sauce. Pour the marinade into a small non-stick saucepan and bring to the boil. Cook for 6 minutes or until the liquid has reduced and the garlic is softened. You need enough of the marinade to pour over the salmon but not swamp it completely.

Put the salmon fillets on warmed plates, carefully lifting off the skin as you go. Spoon the hot sauce over the salmon and serve with a small portion of rice or new potatoes and some steamed or stir-fried vegetables.

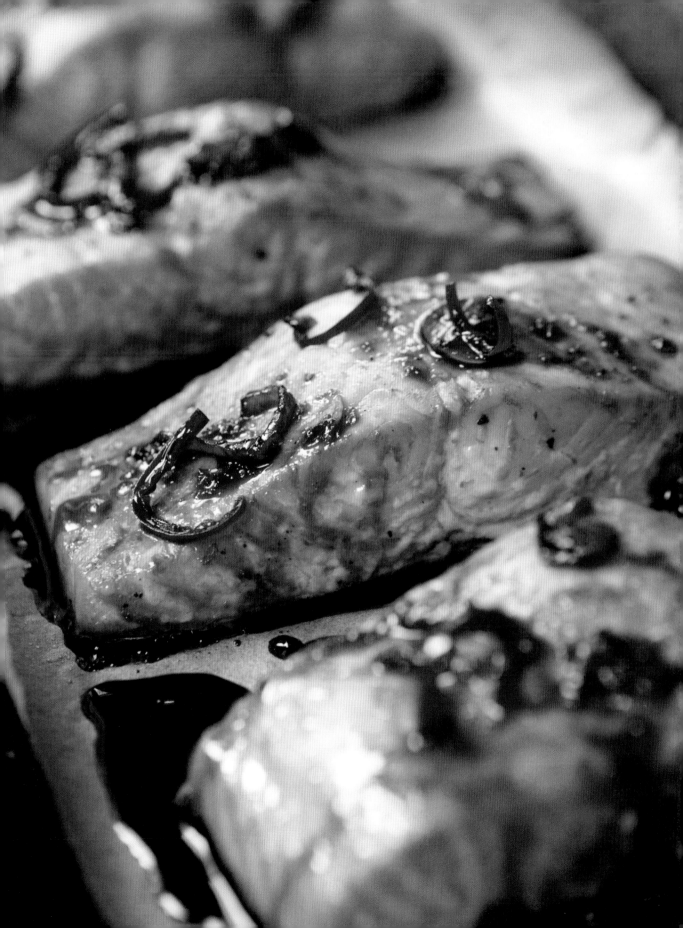

# MASALA-MARINATED CHICKEN WITH MINTED YOGHURT SAUCE

*Dieting or not, this is one of our favourite recipes. It's mouth-wateringly good – the spicy marinade makes the meat really tender and full of flavour, while the yoghurt sauce sets it off a treat. Serve with our cumin-crusted vegetables (see page 108) for a proper spicy feast.*

**SERVES 4–5**

1.65kg chicken
1 lime, quartered
freshly ground black pepper
fresh watercress or baby leaf salad,
to serve

**Marinade**
6 cardamom pods
2 tbsp cumin seeds
2 tbsp coriander seeds
4 whole cloves
1 tsp black peppercorns
1 tsp ground fenugreek
2 tsp ground turmeric
1 tbsp paprika
1–2 tsp hot chilli powder (the more
you use, the spicier the dish)
¼ tsp ground cinnamon
1 tsp flaked sea salt
4 garlic cloves, peeled and crushed
40g chunk of fresh root ginger,
peeled and finely grated
100g low-fat natural yoghurt

**For the minted yoghurt sauce**
200g low-fat natural yoghurt
1 tsp ready-made mint sauce

*320 calories per portion (if serving 4)*
*256 calories per portion (if serving 5)*

To make the marinade, split the cardamom pods and remove the seeds. Put the cardamom seeds in a dry non-stick frying pan and discard the husks. Add the cumin and coriander seeds, cloves and black peppercorns and place the pan over a medium heat. Cook for 1–2 minutes, stirring regularly until the spices are lightly toasted – you know they're ready when you can smell the spicy aroma.

Tip the toasted spices into a pestle and mortar, or an electric spice grinder, and pound to a fine powder. Transfer to a mixing bowl and stir in the fenugreek, turmeric, paprika, chilli powder, cinnamon and salt. Add the garlic, ginger and yoghurt, then mix well and leave to stand while you prepare the chicken.

Place the chicken on its breast on a sturdy chopping board and cut carefully either side of the backbone with good scissors or poultry shears. Chuck out the bone and cut off the foot joints and wing tips.

Strip all the skin off the bird apart from the ends of the wings (which are easier to remove after cooking). You'll find this simpler to do if you snip the membrane between the skin and the chicken flesh as you go. Cut off and discard any obvious fat – it will be a creamy white colour. Open out the chicken and place it on the board so the breast side is facing upwards.

Press down heavily with the palms of your hands to break the breastbone and flatten the chicken as evenly as possible. This will help it cook more quickly. Slash the meat with a knife through the thickest parts of the legs and breasts. Place the chicken in a shallow non-metallic dish – a lasagne dish is ideal – and tuck in the legs and wings.

Spoon over the marinade and really massage it into the chicken on both sides, ensuring that every bit of the bird is well coated – get your hands in there and really go for it. Cover the dish with cling film and put the chicken in the fridge to marinate for at least 4 hours or ideally overnight.

Preheat the oven to 210°C/Fan 190°C/Gas 6½ . Take the chicken out of the dish and place it on a rack inside a large baking tray, breast-side up. Squeeze over some juice from the lime and season with ground black pepper.

Roast for 45–50 minutes until the chicken is lightly browned and cooked throughout, tossing the lime quarters on to the rack for the last 20 minutes to cook alongside the chicken. They'll be good for squeezing over the meat later. The juices should run clear when the thickest part of 1 of the thighs is pierced with a skewer. Cover loosely with foil and leave to rest for 10 minutes before carving.

While the chicken is resting, make the sauce. Spoon the yoghurt into a serving bowl and stir in the mint sauce until thoroughly combined. Transfer the chicken to a plate or wooden board and carve into slices, discarding any skin. Serve with the sauce and some watercress or salad and enjoy!

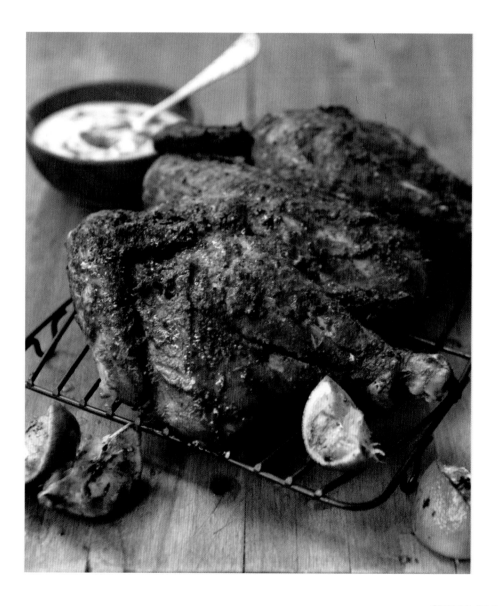

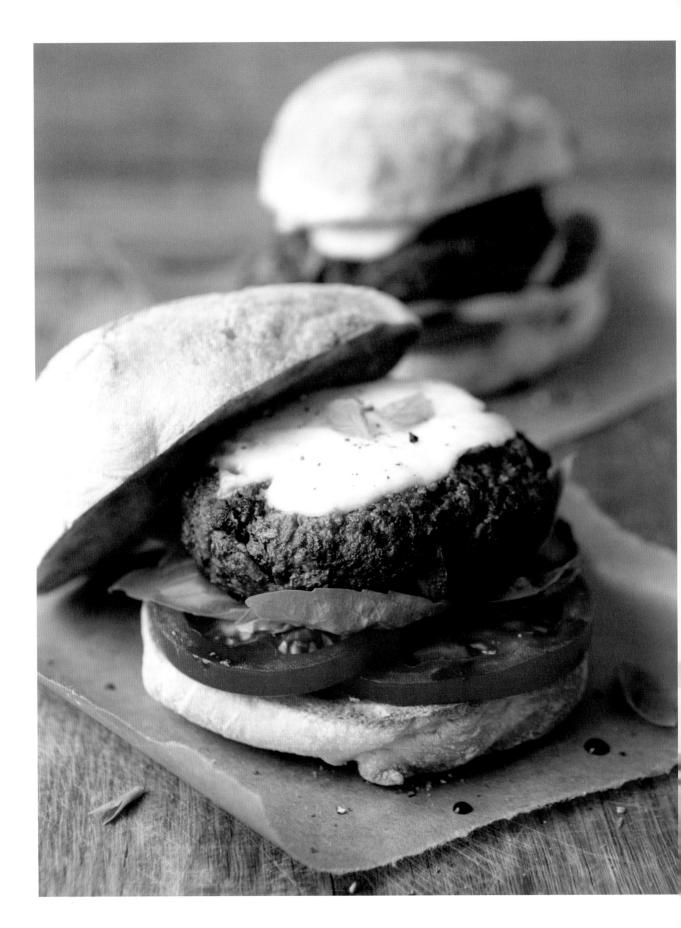

# MEDITERRANEAN BEEF BURGERS

*Everyone loves a burger and you can still eat these when on a diet. Bulking the meat out with some grated onion and courgette makes the burgers feel more generous with few extra calories, and you'll find no one will notice the difference. They'll be too busy enjoying the succulent combination of beef, basil and mozzarella, all packed into crusty ciabatta.*

Trim the courgette and grate it coarsely on to a board, then tip it into a large mixing bowl. Peel the onion and grate it coarsely, then add this to the bowl with the courgette. Put the minced beef, garlic, oregano, basil and tomato paste or purée into the same bowl and season well with salt and pepper. Mix with clean hands until everything is thoroughly combined.

Divide the mince mixture into 4 evenly sized balls and flatten each into a patty shape about 2cm thick. Brush the oil over a large non-stick frying pan and place over a low heat. Fry the burgers gently for about 10 minutes or until nicely browned and cooked through, turning them halfway through the cooking time. Preheat the grill to its hottest setting.

While the burgers are cooking, cut the ciabatta rolls in half horizontally and place them on a grill pan, cut side up. Cook under the preheated grill until lightly toasted. Remove from the heat and take the bread off the tray and put it to one side.

Place the hot burgers on the tray and top each one with a slice of mozzarella. Put the tray back under the grill for another 1–2 minutes or until the mozzarella has melted.

Put the bottom half of each roll on a plate and top with sliced tomatoes and basil leaves. Add a dribble of balsamic vinegar and some black pepper. Add a sizzling hot burger, top with the remaining bread and serve right away. Fantastic!

**SERVES 4**

1 small courgette
1 medium onion
400g lean beef steak mince
2 garlic cloves, peeled and crushed
1 tsp dried oregano
1 tsp dried basil
1 tbsp sun-dried tomato paste or tomato purée
1 tsp sunflower oil
4 ciabatta rolls
100g reduced-fat (light) mozzarella, well drained and cut into 4 slices
2 large ripe vine tomatoes, sliced
fresh basil leaves
balsamic vinegar, for drizzling
fine sea salt
freshly ground black pepper

*413 calories per portion*

*Top tip:* *If you want to reduce the calorie count further, use 2 rolls and serve topless burgers. Calorie count will be just 332 for each.*

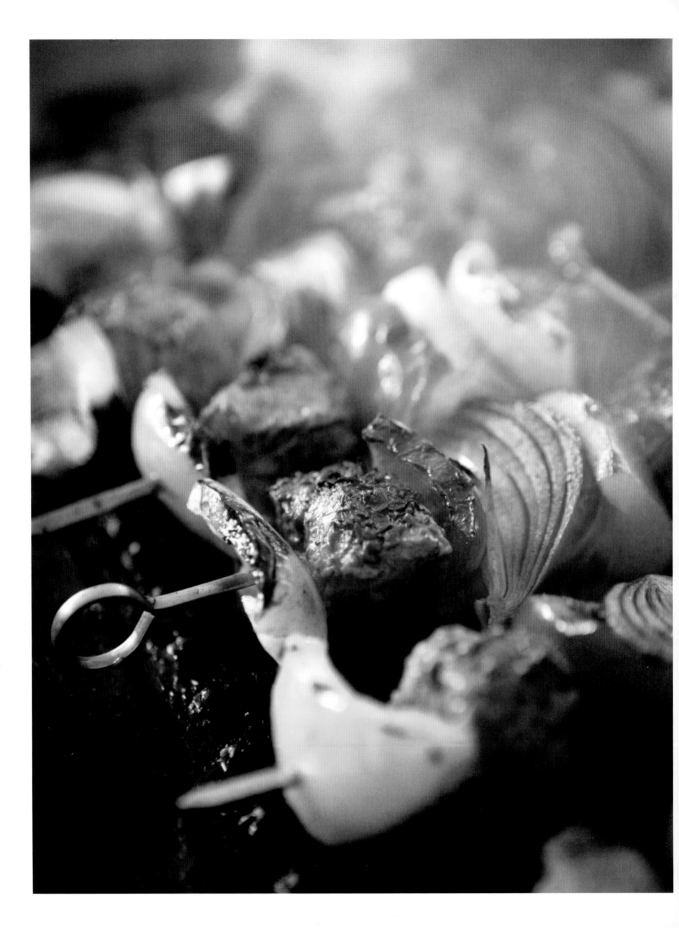

# LEMONY LAMB KEBABS

*There's nothing better than the scent of lemony, herby lamb cooking on the barbecue. It's a healthy way of cooking too, as much of the fat drips away. We like to eat these kebabs tucked into warm pitta bread, but you can also enjoy them with just a side salad or some vegetables.*

To make the marinade, put the cumin, coriander and fennel seeds in a pestle and mortar and pound to a coarse powder. You can use 1½ teaspoon each of ground cumin and coriander if you prefer, but the flavour won't be quite as good as freshly ground spices. Add the thyme leaves and crush them into the spices for a few seconds.

Tip the spices and thyme into a large non-metallic bowl and stir in the lemon zest and juice, garlic, oil, salt and lots of black pepper.

Trim as much fat as possible off the lamb, then cut the meat into rough 3cm chunks – you should have about 40 chunks. Add the lamb to the marinade and toss until well coated. Cover with cling film and chill in the fridge for 30 minutes before cooking.

While the lamb is marinating, prepare the vegetables for the kebabs. Deseed the peppers and cut them into 3cm chunks. Cut each onion into 8 wedges with the root intact.

Remove the lamb from the fridge and thread the meat on to 8 metal skewers – these should be about 25cm long – alternating with the pieces of pepper and onion. Season with a little more salt and pepper.

Cook over a hot barbecue or under a preheated hot grill (close to the element) for 6–8 minutes. Turn once or twice until the lamb and vegetables are lightly charred – the meat should be pink in the middle. Mix the yoghurt, garlic and chopped mint or mint sauce together in a small bowl to make the yoghurt sauce.

Warm the pitta bread on the barbecue, in the toaster or under a grill and carefully cut down one side with a sharp knife. Pull the bread open and stuff with shredded lettuce leaves, grated carrot, tomatoes and cucumber. Slide the meat and vegetables off the skewers and into the pittas using a fork. Drizzle a little of the minty yoghurt sauce and serve with some chilli sauce and lemon wedges too if you fancy.

## MAKES 8 KEBABS

700g lean lamb leg (or leg steaks)
2 small yellow peppers
2 small red peppers
2 small red onions
150ml low-fat natural yoghurt
1 garlic clove, peeled and crushed
1 tbsp finely chopped fresh mint or
1 tsp mint sauce
6 pitta breads
1 romaine lettuce heart, shredded
1 medium carrot, finely grated
3 ripe vine tomatoes, sliced
15cm piece of cucumber,
thinly sliced
flaked sea salt
freshly ground black pepper
lemon wedges and hot chilli sauce,
to serve

### Marinade

2 tsp cumin seeds
2 tsp coriander seeds
1 tsp fennel seeds
1 tbsp fresh thyme leaves
finely grated zest and juice of
1 unwaxed lemon
1 garlic clove, peeled and crushed
1 tbsp extra virgin olive oil
1 tsp fine sea salt
freshly ground black pepper

*203 calories per portion*
*381 calories per portion (with pitta)*

# ROAST PORK WITH APPLE GRAVY

*This pork is flavoured with a delicious lemon, garlic and herb rub. Okay, we know the crackling isn't for anyone watching their weight, but it really does keep the pork beautifully moist as it cooks and you can let the others eat it. Serve with our special apple gravy and lots of roasted peppers, courgettes and onions.*

**SERVES 6**

1.25kg loin of pork with deeply scored rind
10g fresh sage leaves
15g flat-leaf parsley
finely grated zest of 1 unwaxed lemon
4 garlic cloves, crushed
1 tsp flaked sea salt
freshly ground black pepper

**Apple gravy**
200ml apple juice (preferably the cloudy type)
125ml cold water
2 tsp cornflour
freshly ground black pepper

*263 calories per portion (without crackling)*

Put the pork on a board and cut off the string if your pork has been rolled and tied. Slide a large sharp knife under the pork rind and fat, then lift it off completely. Set it to one side. Cut a hole about 4cm wide through the thickest part of the loin, or eye, of the pork. Preheat the oven to 190°C/Fan 170°C/Gas 5.

Finely chop the sage and parsley leaves and put them in a bowl. Add the lemon zest, garlic, salt and plenty of freshly ground black pepper. Press some of this herby mix into the hole in the pork and then spread the rest over the surface of the pork until well covered.

Cover the meat with the pork rind – this will protect the pork and keep it moist as it cooks. Tie the joint at 2cm intervals with kitchen string to keep it together and place in a small sturdy roasting tin. Roast for 30 minutes per 500g, plus 20 minutes. A 1.25kg joint should take 1 hour 35 minutes, but check it is cooked throughout.

When the pork is ready, move it to a warmed board ready to carve and cover it with foil and a couple of dry tea towels to keep it warm. Holding the roasting tin carefully with an oven cloth, tilt all the juices to one corner and skim off as much of that naughty fat as possible with a spoon and throw it out.

To make the gravy, put the roasting tin on the hob over a medium heat and add the apple juice and 50ml of the cold water. Stir well to lift the juices and sediment from the bottom of the pan. Simmer for a couple of minutes. Carefully strain the gravy through a sieve into a small saucepan and bring it back to a simmer. Mix the cornflour and the remaining cold water to make a thin paste. Stir this into the gravy and cook for 1–2 minutes more until thickened, stirring occasionally. Adjust the seasoning to taste.

Remove the string from the pork and lift off the crackling and cut it up separately. Carve the pork and serve it without the crackling for anyone watching their weight! Pour the gravy into a jug to serve with the pork.

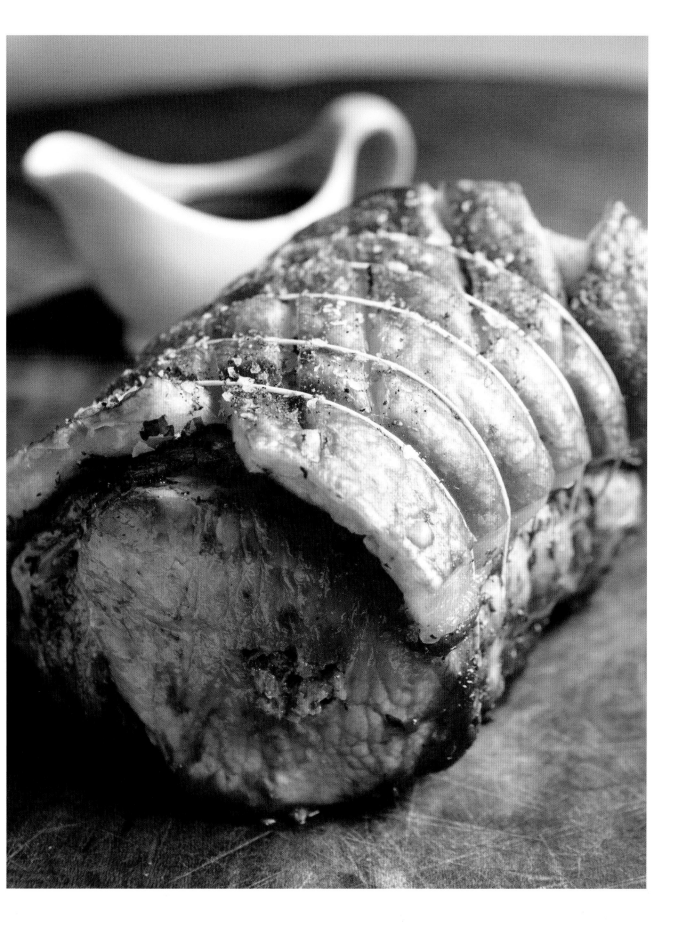

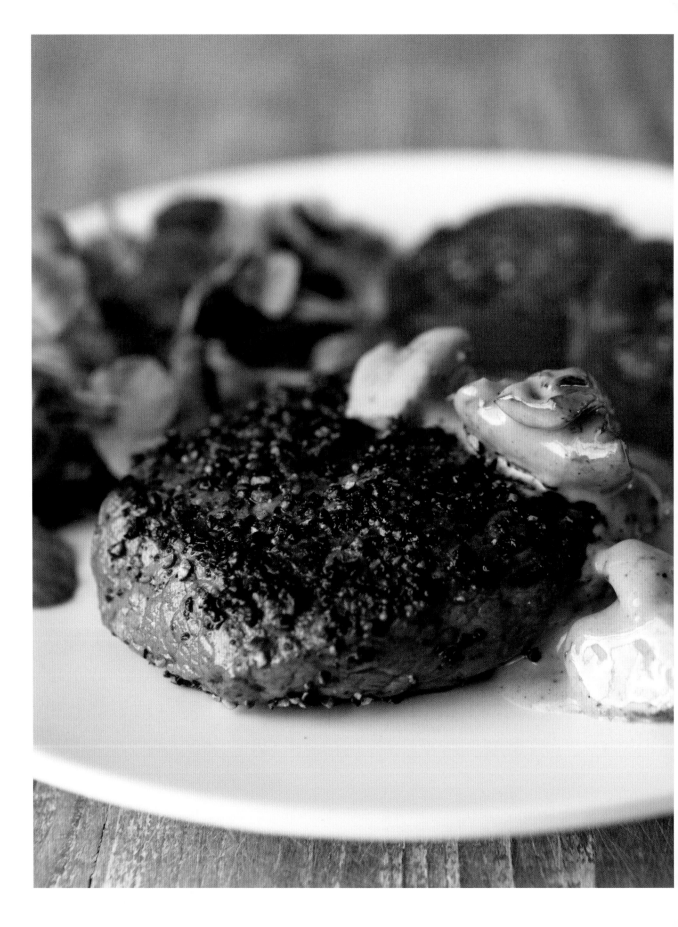

# PEPPERED STEAK WITH MUSHROOMS

*What could be better than a good steak with creamy mushrooms? And despite the rich taste the sauce isn't too high in fat. We like rump steak, but use fillet if you prefer and cook for 3–4 minutes on each side. If you don't have a pestle and mortar, use a pepper grinder for the peppercorns.*

Put the steak on a board and cut off all the hard fat. Cut the steak in half to give 2 portions – each should weigh about 140g by the time you've trimmed off the fat. Put the peppercorns in a pestle and mortar and pound until coarsely ground. Stir in the salt.

Pour a teaspoon of the oil into a small dish or eggcup, dip the end of a pastry brush in the oil and brush the steaks on both sides. Coat the steaks generously with the pepper and salt mixture.

Cut the tomatoes in half and place them on a grill pan lined with foil, cut side up. Season the tomatoes with a little ground black pepper, then cook under a preheated hot grill for 5–8 minutes until softened.

Pour the remaining oil into a small non-stick frying pan. Place over a high heat and stir-fry the mushrooms for 2–3 minutes until lightly browned. Make sure you keep the heat up high so they get some lovely colour. Tip the mushrooms into a bowl and return the pan to a medium-high heat.

Put the steaks in the pan and cook for 2–3 minutes on each side or according to taste. Two minutes on each side should give you a medium-rare steak.

Put the steaks on warmed plates and leave them to rest. Return the mushrooms to the pan and warm through over a high heat. Dissolve the stock in the just-boiled water and add to the pan, stirring constantly to lift the sediment and juices from the bottom of the pan.

Add the crème fraiche, mustard and wine, if using, and stir together for 1–2 minutes until the sauce is hot and has thickened slightly. Spoon the mushrooms and sauce over the steaks and serve with the grilled tomatoes and a large, lightly dressed salad.

**SERVES 2**

1 lean rump steak (about 325g), 2cm thick
1 tbsp black peppercorns, plus extra to season
½ tsp flaked sea salt, plus extra to season
1 tbsp sunflower oil
2 large ripe vine tomatoes
75g small chestnut mushrooms, wiped and halved (or quartered if large)
¼ beef stock cube
150ml just-boiled water
3 tbsp half-fat crème fraiche
½ tsp Dijon mustard
2 tbsp white wine (optional)

*308 calories per portion*

# GAMMON WITH PARSLEY SAUCE

*This is a low-fat version of a classic dish that is one of our all-time favourites. Making the parsley sauce with cornflour instead of butter keeps it low in fat, but it's still really tasty. If you don't believe us, try it for yourself. Pineapple rings optional!*

**SERVES 4**

1 tsp sunflower oil
4 gammon steaks (smoked or unsmoked)
freshly ground black pepper

**Parsley sauce**
300ml semi-skimmed milk
1 small onion, quartered
1 bay leaf
10g cornflour (about 1½ tbsp)
2 tbsp cold water
3 heaped tbsp finely chopped parsley (curly parsley works best here)
flaked sea salt
freshly ground black pepper

*334 calories per portion (without potatoes and beans)*

To make the sauce, put the milk, onion and bay leaf in a medium saucepan and bring to a gentle simmer. Take off the heat and leave to stand for 10 minutes. Use tongs or a slotted spoon to remove the onion and bay leaf and throw them away.

Brush a large non-stick frying pan with the sunflower oil and place it over a medium-high heat. Snip the gammon fat off completely with a pair of kitchen scissors. Season the gammon with ground black pepper, then cook the steaks for 2½–3 minutes on each side. If your pan isn't large enough for all the gammon steaks together, cook a couple and keep them warm in a low oven while you do the rest.

While the gammon is cooking, place the pan with the infused milk over a medium heat and stir in the parsley. In a small bowl, mix the cornflour with the cold water until smooth and pour into the pan with the milk. Heat through, stirring constantly until the sauce is smooth and thick. Season to taste.

Put the gammon steaks on warmed plates. Pour over a little of the sauce and serve the rest separately. We like serving this gammon with a few new potatoes and some freshly cooked runner beans.

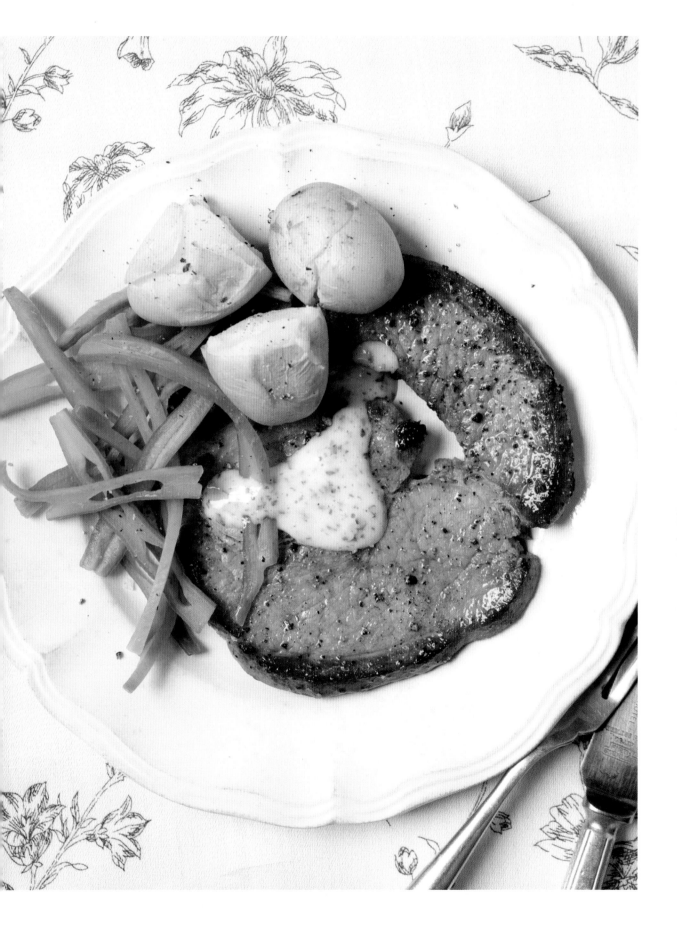

# LEMON AND THYME ROAST CHICKEN

*A good roast chicken is one of our favourite meals and by adding lemon and thyme to flavour the meat you don't miss the stuffing. Even though we're watching our weight we can still enjoy a chicken dinner, but now we don't eat the skin – contains loads of calories, we're told.*

**SERVES 5–6**

1 free-range roasting chicken (about 1.75kg)
4 bushy sprigs of thyme or 1 tsp dried thyme
½ large lemon
1 medium onion, peeled and sliced
4 rashers of rindless dry-cure smoked back bacon
flaked sea salt
freshly ground black pepper

**Gravy**
100ml white wine (or extra chicken stock)
300ml chicken stock, made with ½ chicken stock cube
1 tbsp redcurrant jelly
2 rashers of rindless dry-cure smoked back bacon
2 tsp cornflour
1 tbsp cold water

*362 calories per portion (if serving 5)*
*302 calories per portion (if serving 6)*

Preheat the oven to 190°C/Fan 170°C/Gas 5. Remove any elastic bands that may be trussing the chicken. Put the chicken on a board and slide your fingers under the skin of the breast, carefully separating it from the flesh. This is much easier than it sounds, so just go for it. Gently push the thyme sprigs up under the chicken skin – the idea is to add some extra flavour to the meat. Squeeze the lemon all over the bird and rub the juice into the chicken skin.

Pile the onion slices in the centre of a sturdy roasting tin and place the chicken on top. Don't allow any onion to escape around the outside of the chicken as it may burn. Pop the squeezed lemon half inside the chicken, then wash your hands and season the bird with sea salt and plenty of black pepper. Roast in the centre of the oven for 45 minutes per 1 kilogram, plus 20 minutes – a 1.75kg chicken will take about 1 hour 35 minutes.

Half an hour before the end of the cooking time, take the chicken out of the oven and cover the breast with the 4 bacon rashers. Put the tin back in the oven until the chicken is thoroughly cooked. The juices should run clear when the thigh is pieced with a skewer and there should be no pink remaining.

Move the chicken and bacon to a warmed serving dish and scoop up any onions that you are able to lift from the pan and place them on the dish as well. Cover the chicken with foil and a couple of dry tea towels and leave it to rest. Holding the roasting tin carefully with an oven cloth, tilt all the juices to one corner. Skim as much fat from the surface as possible and chuck it away.

To make the gravy, put the roasting tin on the hob over a medium heat and pour in the wine and stock. Stir well to lift the juices and sediment from the bottom of the pan – these will add lots of flavour to the gravy – and bring to a simmer. Pour the gravy carefully into a medium saucepan and add the 2 remaining rashers of bacon. Bring to a gentle simmer and cook for 5 minutes, stirring occasionally. The bacon adds extra flavour to the gravy.

Take the bacon rashers out of the pan with tongs or a fork and put them with the rest. Mix the cornflour with the water in a small bowl and stir it into the gravy. Heat through until bubbling and simmer for a further minute, stirring until thickened. Strain the gravy through a fine sieve into a warmed jug.

Carve the chicken and serve it on warmed plates, adding a little of the roasted onion and a rasher of bacon to each one. Pour over a little of the gravy and serve the rest separately.

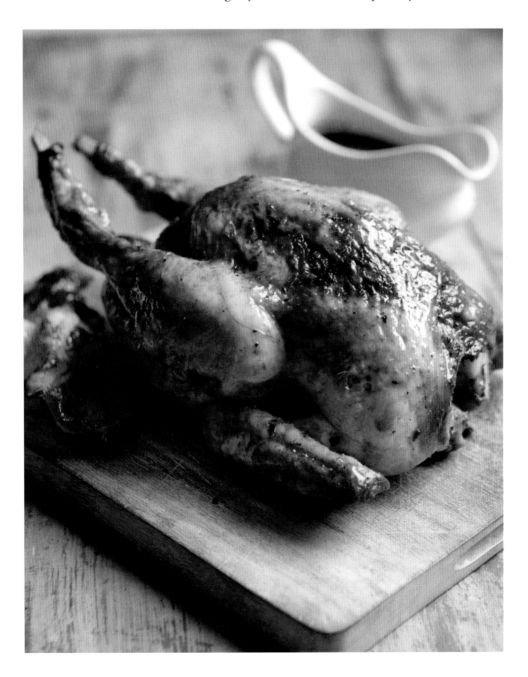

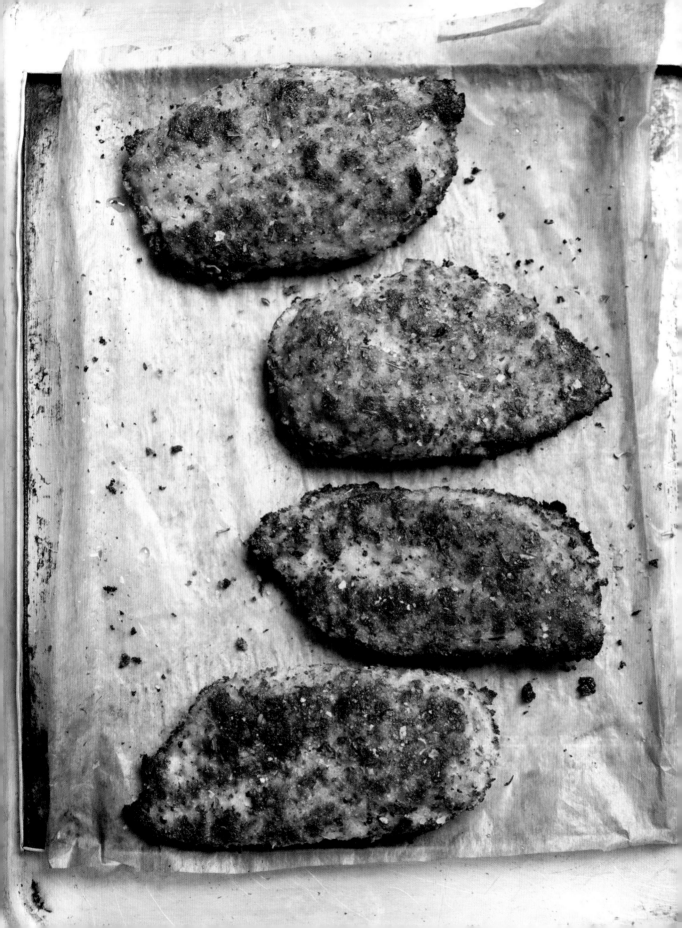

# EASY CRISPY CHICKEN

*This is finger-licking good and all the family will love it – they won't even realise how low in calories it is! If you like, you can use 100g ready-made white breadcrumbs instead of making your own.*

Preheat the oven to 220°C/Fan 200°C/Gas 7. Place the bread on a large baking tray lined with baking parchment and toast until pale golden brown. Leave to cool for 5 minutes, then remove the crusts and tear the bread into large pieces.

Put the bread in a food processor and blitz into crumbs. Tip these into a large bowl and toss with the oregano, salt and Parmesan cheese, then season with lots of black pepper. Divide the crumb mixture between 2 dinner plates. Spoon the yoghurt into a bowl and sprinkle the flour on a plate.

Take a chicken breast and coat it lightly in the flour, shaking off any excess, then dip it into the yoghurt until evenly covered. Then place the chicken on a plate of crumb mix and press so you get a thickish crust all over.

Transfer the chicken carefully to the lined baking tray. Continue dipping and coating the rest of the chicken breasts until they all have a lovely crust of crumbs. Each plate of crumbs should be enough to coat 2 breasts.

Bake the chicken for 22–25 minutes until golden, crisp and cooked through. Leave to stand for 4–5 minutes before serving with some fresh green salad.

**SERVES 4**

150g white sliced bread (about 4 slices)
4 tsp dried oregano or dried mixed herbs
2 tsp flaked sea salt
25g Parmesan cheese, finely grated
4 tbsp low-fat natural yoghurt
1–2 tbsp plain flour
4 boneless, skinless chicken breasts (each about 160g)
freshly ground black pepper

*299 calories per portion*

*Top tip:* *To make the chicken extra crispy, as in our photo, spray with a spritz of sunflower oil before baking.*

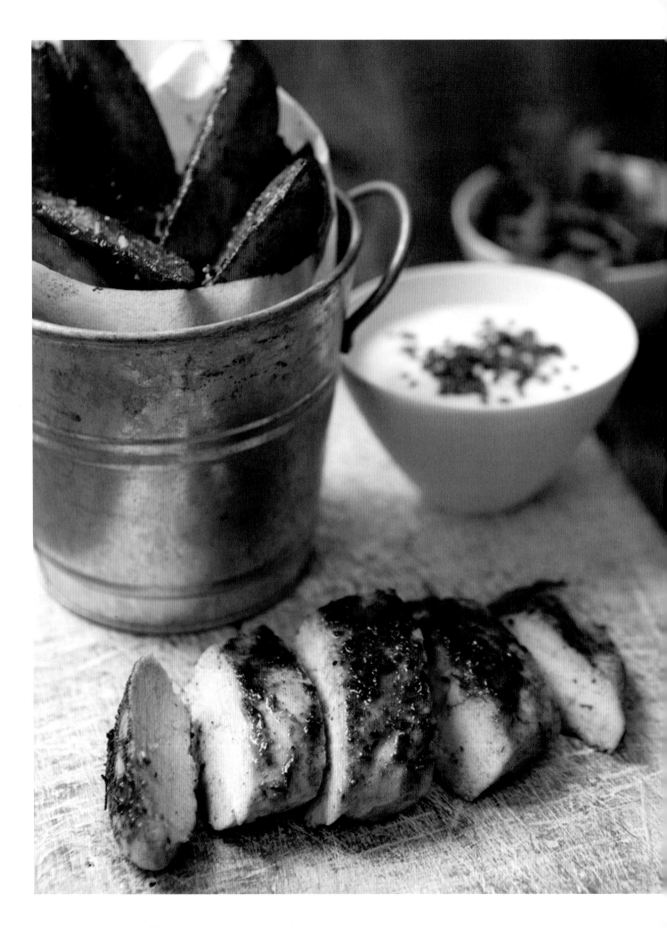

# CAJUN SPICED CHICKEN WITH POTATO WEDGES AND CHIVE DIP

*This recipe, with its raging Cajun spicy flavours, was inspired by the fab food we ate when we made our trip down the Mississippi. It's a real treat but surprisingly low in fat, so you can enjoy a few – and we mean a few – potato wedges alongside.*

Preheat the oven to 220°C/Fan 200°C/Gas 7. To make the Cajun spice mix, put the spices and salt in a jar and seal tightly with a screw-top lid. Give the jar a really good shake so that all the spices are mixed together – you can do a bit of a samba at the same time! This spice mix can now be stored in a cool, dark place for several weeks.

Peel the potatoes and cut them into 8–10 long wedges, depending on how big they are, and put them in a bowl. Add the oil and toss lightly to coat all the wedges. Sprinkle with the paprika, salt and lots of freshly ground black pepper, then scatter them on to a baking tray. Cook in the preheated oven for 20–25 minutes, until tender and lightly browned.

While the potatoes are cooking, place each chicken breast between 2 sheets of cling film and beat with a rolling pin until the meat is about 1.5cm thick. You need to make the chicken breasts all the same thickness so they cook evenly.

Brush a griddle pan or non-stick frying pan with a little oil and place over a medium-high heat until hot. Sprinkle 1 teaspoon of the spice mix over each chicken breast to dust it lightly.

Griddle or pan-fry the chicken breasts for 2 minutes, then turn them over with tongs and cook on the other side for a further 2 minutes. Finish by cooking the chicken for 1 more minute on each side or until cooked through. There should be no pink remaining. Put the chicken breasts on a plate and leave them to rest for 3–4 minutes.

To make the chive dip, mix the yoghurt and chives together. Spoon into small pots and put 1 on each plate. Divide the potato wedges between the plates and add the cooked chicken breasts. Serve with lime wedges for squeezing over the chicken and a large mixed salad.

## SERVES 4

4 boneless, skinless chicken breasts
½ tsp sunflower oil, for greasing
lime wedges, to serve

**Cajun spice mix**
5 tsp ground cumin
4 tsp smoked paprika
2 tsp dried thyme
2 tsp dried oregano
2 tsp coarsely ground black pepper
½ tsp cayenne pepper
1 tsp flaked sea salt

**Potato wedges**
3 medium potatoes (about 475g)
1 tsp sunflower oil
½ tsp paprika
½ tsp flaked sea salt
freshly ground black pepper

**Chive dip**
100g low-fat natural yoghurt
2 tbsp finely chopped chives

*284 calories per portion*

# HARISSA CHICKEN WITH BULGUR WHEAT SALAD

*This is a lovely light but tasty recipe and the chicken is brightened up no end by a touch of spicy harissa paste. Harissa comes from North Africa and is a mixture of peppers, dried chillies, garlic, cumin and other spices. It's great as a marinade or for adding a fiery touch to sauces, meat or fish. Our favourite is rose harissa, which includes rose petals among its ingredients and is available in lots of supermarkets.*

**SERVES 4**

4 boneless, skinless chicken breasts
½ tsp sunflower oil
1 tbsp harissa paste (preferably
rose harissa)
lemon wedges, to serve

**Bulgur wheat salad**
100g bulgur wheat
150g cherry tomatoes, halved or
quartered if large
¼ cucumber, diced
4 spring onions, trimmed
and finely sliced
1 garlic clove, peeled and crushed
small bunch of flat-leaf parsley
(about 10g), plus extra to garnish
small bunch of fresh mint
(about 10g)
finely grated zest of ½
unwaxed lemon
freshly squeezed juice of ½ lemon
freshly ground black pepper

*270 calories per portion*

To make the salad, rinse the bulgur wheat in a fine sieve and tip it into a medium saucepan. Cover with cold water and bring to the boil, then cook for about 10 minutes until just tender, or follow the packet instructions. Rinse the bulgur in a sieve under running water until cold and leave to drain.

Tip the cooked bulgur wheat into a large serving bowl and add the tomatoes, cucumber, spring onions, garlic, parsley, mint, lemon zest and juice. You'll need about 3 heaped tablespoons of each herb once chopped. Season with lots of freshly ground black pepper, toss everything together well and leave to stand while you cook the chicken.

Place each chicken breast between 2 sheets of cling film and beat with a rolling pin until about 1.5cm thick. You need to make the chicken breasts about the same thickness so they cook evenly.

Brush a griddle pan or non-stick frying pan with a little oil and place over a medium-high heat until hot. Griddle or pan-fry the chicken breasts for 2 minutes, then turn them over with tongs and cook on the other side for another 2 minutes.

Brush the chicken breasts with half of the harissa on 1 side only and turn over. Cook for a minute while brushing the reverse side with the remaining harissa. Flip over and cook for a further minute or until cooked through. Check that there is no pinkness remaining.

Transfer the chicken to a board and leave to rest for 3–4 minutes before serving. Garnish with extra parsley and the lemon wedges and serve hot with the bulgur salad.

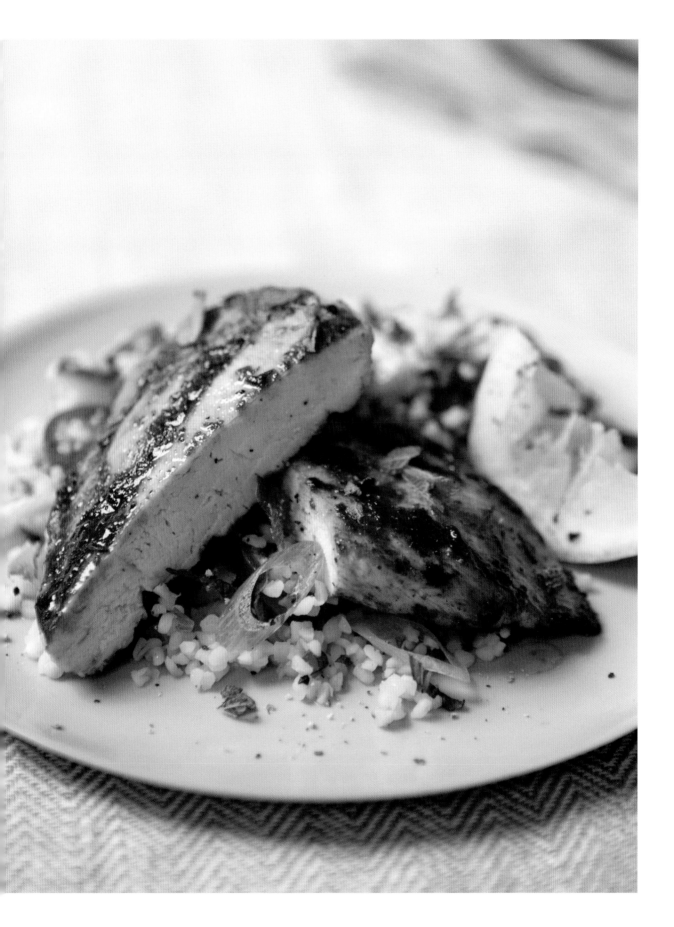

# SI AND DAVE'S WEIGHT-LOSS TIPS

———

A gratin topping, made with breadcrumbs and grated cheese, is lighter than a pastry crust or buttery mash and still makes a tasty pie.

———

Another idea is to use a topping of scrunched-up filo pastry, which is deliciously crisp and crunchy but low in fat.

———

Our favourite trick is to make a fab lasagne, replacing the carb-heavy pasta with sheets of leek. It's amazing.

———

We couldn't give up our pies but we've found out how to make a clever pastry with pizza base mix. No fat needed.

———

If you make cottage pie, use lean beef, not extra-lean because it's too dry, and bulk out the mash with some sliced leeks.

———

Make sure you trim any visible fat off the meat you use for your pies.

———

Add any condiments you like. Ketchup, brown sauce, mustards, pickles and chutneys aren't calorie free, but the small amount added to your meal won't ruin your weight loss.

———

# PIES

"A good trick – use smaller plates. Makes it look and feel like you've got more food!"

*Si*

# QUICK COD AND PRAWN GRATIN

*Everyone loves a fish pie and this is a lighter than usual version, with a crunchy breadcrumb and cheese topping rather than mashed potatoes. It's quick to make too and ready to eat in under 20 minutes. We like to use extra-mature Cheddar, as its strong flavour means a little goes a long way.*

### SERVES 4

100g frozen cooked peeled prawns
400g thick white fish fillet, such as line-caught cod, skinned
150g smoked haddock, skinned
400ml semi-skimmed milk
1 bay leaf
½ small onion, finely chopped
3 tbsp cornflour
3 tbsp cold water
100g frozen peas
2 tbsp white wine or vermouth
40g dry white breadcrumbs, ideally fairly coarse
25g extra-mature Cheddar, finely grated
flaked sea salt
freshly ground black pepper

*287 calories per portion*

Spread the prawns on a plate and leave them to thaw at room temperature while you prepare the rest of the ingredients. Cut the white fish fillet and haddock into 3cm chunks and set them aside. Pour the milk into a large non-stick saucepan and add the bay leaf and onion, then bring to a gentle simmer.

Mix the cornflour and water together in a small bowl until smooth, then pour this into the warm milk. Cook over a low heat for 5 minutes, stirring constantly with a wooden spoon until the sauce is thick, smooth and bubbling gently and the onion is tender. Season with salt and pepper.

Stir the peas and white wine (or vermouth) into the hot sauce and cook for 1 minute, stirring constantly. Add the fish pieces and cook for 2 minutes more, stirring once or twice. Stir the prawns, with any water released from them as they thawed, into the sauce and cook for another 2 minutes or until the prawns are hot and the fish is cooked. Stir only occasionally so the fish doesn't break up too much – you want your finished gratin to be nice and chunky.

Preheat the grill to its hottest setting. Spoon the fish mixture into a warmed 1.5-litre shallow pie dish. Mix the breadcrumbs and cheese together and sprinkle them over the top. Place under the grill for 2–3 minutes or until the cheese has melted and the breadcrumbs are lightly toasted. Serve piping hot with some green vegetables.

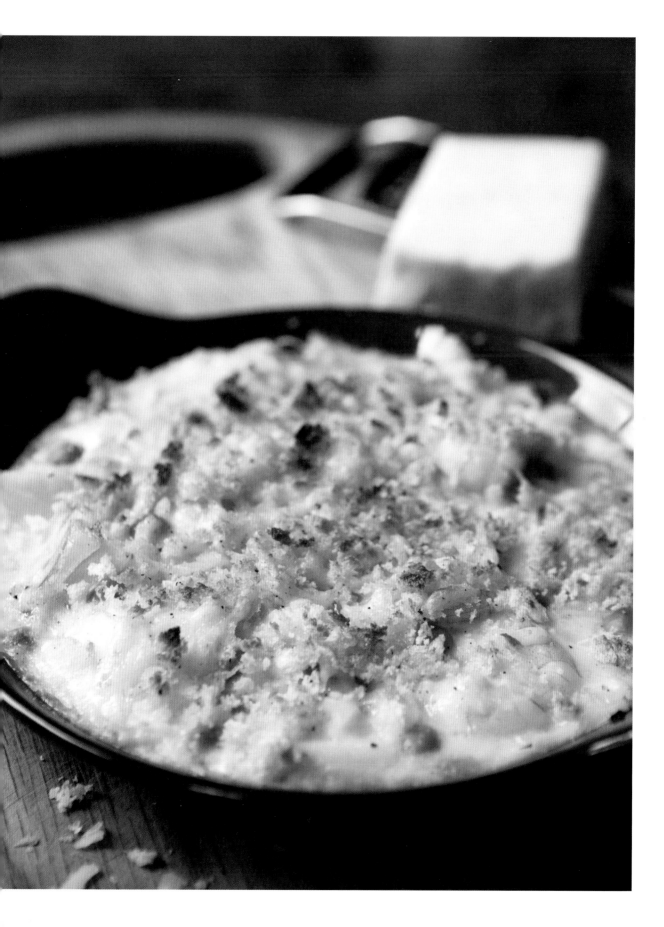

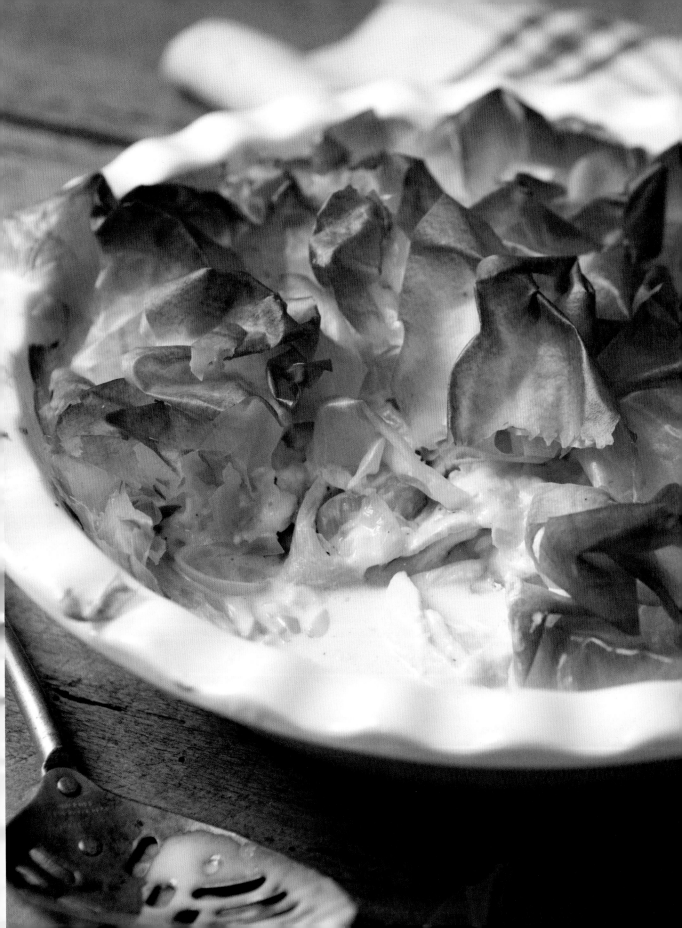

# CHICKEN AND HAM
# TANGLE PIE

*Pastry is generally out of bounds when you're dieting, but this scrunchy filo topping is much lower in calories than a regular pastry lid. The pie tastes so rich and creamy you can hardly believe how little fat it contains – try it and we know you'll agree with us.*

Heat the oil in a large non-stick frying pan over a low heat and add the onion and crushed garlic. Fry gently for 5 minutes until the onion is softened, but not coloured, stirring occasionally. Add the leek and cook for 1 minute more, stirring constantly.

Pour over the white wine and 100ml of the water. Dissolve the stock cube in the pan by squishing it with a wooden spoon. Keep simmering on a high heat and stir constantly until the liquid has reduced by about half, then remove the pan from the heat.

Strip off the skin from the chicken and tear the meat off the bones and into bite-sized pieces. Place them in a large bowl. Cut the ham into strips about 1.5cm wide and add them to the bowl. Sprinkle the flour on top and toss lightly together.

Add the onion and stock mixture, the rest of the water and the crème fraiche. Season with lots of freshly ground black pepper and stir all the ingredients together until just combined. Spoon into a 1.5-litre pie dish. Preheat the oven to 200°C/Fan 180°C/Gas 6.

Pile the filo sheets on the work surface, one on top of the other, and divide into 9 rectangles, cutting through all the layers. Put the oil into a small bowl.

One at a time, brush each pastry rectangle lightly with a little oil and very loosely scrunch it up. You'll need to just dip the tip of the pastry brush in the oil to make sure the oil lasts for all the pastry. Place the scrunched-up filo on top of the filling, putting the pieces close together until the surface of the pie is completely covered.

Bake the pie for 30–35 minutes or until the pastry is crisp and golden brown and the filling is bubbling. Serve with some green vegetables – no need to add extra potatoes or rice.

**SERVES 5**

2 tsp sunflower oil
1 medium onion, peeled and finely chopped
2 garlic cloves, peeled and crushed
1 medium leek, trimmed and cut into thin slices
100ml white wine
150ml water
1 chicken stock cube
1kg whole cooked chicken
100g sliced smoked ham
2 tbsp plain flour
300g half-fat crème fraiche
freshly ground black pepper

**Pastry**
3 sheets filo pastry, each about 38 x 30cm
1½–2½ tsp sunflower oil

*429 calories per portion*

**Top tip:** *If you can't get hold of a whole chicken, use about 500g of cooked chicken breast meat instead.*

# SKINNY BEEF LASAGNE

*Who would have thought you could eat lasagne when on a diet? Well, thanks to our amazingly clever recipe, you can. The pasta is replaced with sheets of blanched leeks so you have all the deliciousness without the high calorie count. Fools your eyes as well as your belly – magic!*

**SERVES 6**

2 large leeks, each about 300g
1 medium onion
2 celery sticks, trimmed
2 smallish carrots, peeled
500g lean minced beef
2 garlic cloves, peeled and crushed
150g chestnut mushrooms, wiped and chopped
2 tbsp plain flour
150ml red wine
400ml beef stock, made with 1 beef stock cube
400g can of chopped tomatoes
2 tbsp tomato purée
1 heaped tsp dried oregano
2 bay leaves
500ml semi-skimmed milk
3 tbsp cornflour
freshly grated nutmeg, to taste
50g extra-mature Cheddar, grated
25g Parmesan, finely grated
3 medium vine tomatoes, sliced
freshly ground black pepper

*354 calories per portion*

Trim the leeks until they are about the same width as your lasagne dish. Cut the leeks lengthways through to the middle but no further. Open out and remove 5 or 6 of the narrow leaves from the centre of each leek. Thinly slice these inner leaves. Separate the larger leaves – these will become your 'lasagne'. Finely chop half the onion and cut the other half into wedges. Thinly slice the celery and dice the carrots.

Put the minced beef in a large non-stick frying pan or sauté pan with the sliced leeks, chopped onion, celery, carrots and garlic. Place over a medium-high heat and fry without added fat for about 10 minutes until lightly coloured. You'll need to break up the mince with a couple of wooden spatulas or spoons as it cooks. Stir in the chopped mushrooms and cook for 2–3 minutes more. The pan should look fairly dry at this point.

Sprinkle over the plain flour and stir it thoroughly into the mince and vegetables. Slowly stir in the red wine and stock. Add the canned tomatoes, tomato purée and dried oregano, then drop a bay leaf into the pan and bring it to a simmer. Season with lots of freshly ground black pepper. Turn down the heat slightly and leave the mince to simmer for 20–30 minutes until rich and thick, stirring occasionally.

While the mince is cooking, put the onion wedges in a saucepan with the remaining bay leaf. Mix 3 tablespoons of the milk with the cornflour in a small bowl. Pour the rest of the milk into the pan with the onion wedges and set it over a low heat. Bring to a very gentle simmer and cook for 2–3 minutes. Remove from the heat and leave the milk to infuse for 10 minutes.

Half fill a large saucepan with water and bring to the boil. Add the leek 'lasagne' and bring the water back to the boil. Cook for 5 minutes or until very tender. It is important that the leeks are tender or the lasagne will be tricky to cut later. Drain in a colander under running water until cold. Drain on kitchen paper or a clean tea towel.

Preheat the oven to 200°C/Fan 180°C/Gas 6. Remove the onion wedges and bay leaf from the infused milk with a slotted spoon, then return the pan to the heat. Give the cornflour and milk mixture a good stir until it is smooth once more and pour it into the pan with the infused milk.

Bring to a simmer and cook for 5 minutes, stirring regularly with a silicone whisk until the sauce is smooth and thick. Season with a good grating of nutmeg to taste and plenty of ground black pepper. If the sauce is a little too thick to pour easily, whisk in a couple more tablespoons of milk.

Spoon a third of the mince mixture into a 2.5-litre lasagne dish. Top with a layer of blanched leeks. Repeat the layers twice more, finishing with leeks. Pour the white sauce over the leeks and top with the sliced tomatoes. Mix the Cheddar and Parmesan cheese and sprinkle all over the top. Bake for 30 minutes or until golden brown and bubbling.

Divide into portions with your sharpest knife. Serve with a freshly dressed green salad.

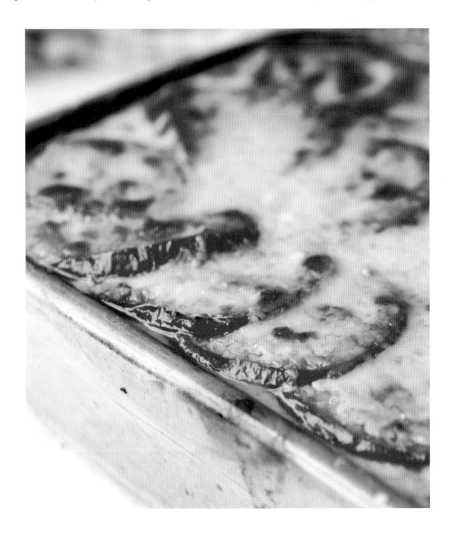

# LOW-FAT MINCED BEEF AND POTATO PIES

*As you all know, we love our pies and we hated the idea of giving them up while we're trying to lose weight. Fortunately, we got this idea for a low-fat 'pastry' cases from our clever friend Justine and meat pies are back on the menu. You'll need some small individual foil pie dishes.*

**MAKES 6**

1 medium onion, finely diced
2 small carrots, peeled and diced
2 celery sticks, trimmed and finely sliced
250g lean minced beef (less than 10% fat)
1 tbsp tomato ketchup
1 tbsp brown sauce
½ tbsp Worcestershire sauce
1 tbsp plain flour
½ tsp hot chilli powder
½ tsp dried chilli flakes (optional)
½ tsp freshly ground black pepper
200g floury potatoes, preferably King Edwards or Maris Pipers, peeled and cut into 1.5cm cubes
300ml beef stock, made with 1 beef stock cube
75g frozen peas

**Pastry**
2 x 145g packets of pizza base mix
about 200ml lukewarm water
plain flour, for kneading and rolling
1–2 tbsp semi-skimmed milk

*335 calories per portion*

Put the onion, carrots, celery and beef together in a large non-stick saucepan and dry-fry over a high heat for 2–3 minutes, until the beef is no longer pink. Keep stirring with a couple of wooden spoons to break up the mince.

Reduce the heat and add the ketchup, brown sauce, Worcestershire sauce, flour, chilli powder and chilli flakes (if using) and black pepper. Cook for 1 minute, then add the potatoes and stock. Bring to the boil, reduce the heat and cover loosely. Simmer for 25 minutes until the potatoes are tender, stirring occasionally. If necessary, remove the lid for the last 5 minutes and stir more regularly until the mixture is thick. Remove from the heat, stir in the frozen peas and leave to cool completely.

To make the pastry, put the pizza base mixes in a large bowl and mix with lukewarm water according to the packet instructions. Turn out on to a lightly floured surface and knead for 5 minutes until the dough is smooth and elastic. Preheat the oven to 200°C/ Fan 180°C/Gas 6.

Using scales, divide the dough into 6 even portions – each will be about 80g. From each portion, take off 35g of the dough to use for the pie lids. Roll out the larger piece of each portion on a lightly floured surface until it is about 3mm thick and large enough to line your foil pie dish, leaving a little overhanging the sides. Lift into a pie dish and press down well into the base and sides. This can be a little tricky first time round, but the dough is very forgiving, so take it slowly until you've got the hang of the method.

Spoon a sixth of the mince and potato mixture into the pie case. Brush the overhanging edges with a little milk. Roll out the smaller portion of pastry until it is large enough to cover the pie dish. Lift it on top of the pie and pinch the pastry firmly together. Trim with kitchen scissors – using scissors will stop the dough stretching.

Repeat exactly the same process to make the other 5 pies and place them on a baking tray. Snip once in the centre of each pastry lid with scissors to create a large hole for steam to escape. Brush the pies generously with more milk.

Bake the pies for 15 minutes, then remove them from the oven and cover each one fairly tightly with foil. Put them back in the oven for a further 15 minutes or until the pies are pale golden brown and the filling is piping hot. Leave to stand for 5 minutes before removing the foil, then tuck in!

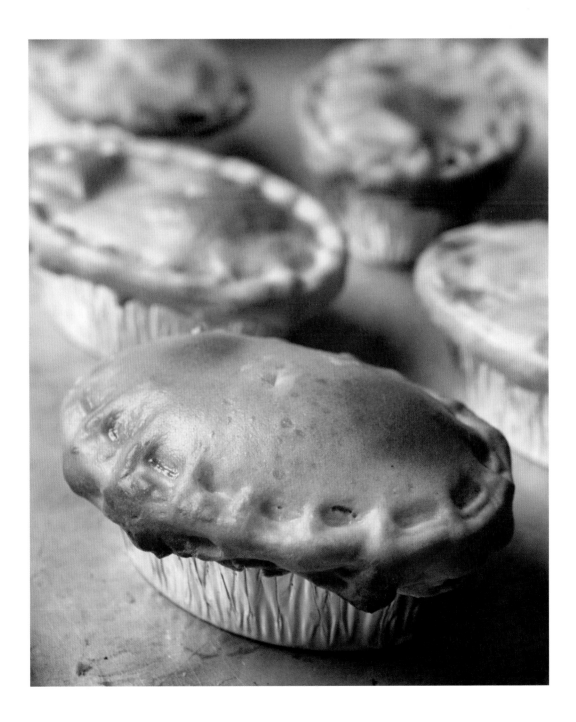

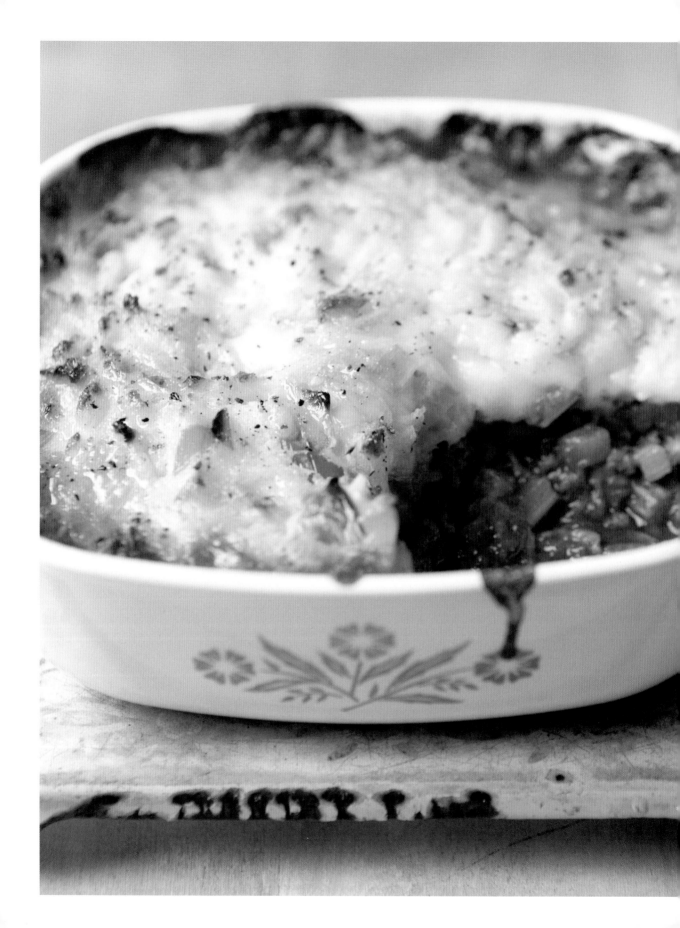

# COTTAGE PIE

*Cottage pie is a hearty dish and one that we love to eat. Happily, this version is lower in calories than usual so we can continue to enjoy one of our favourite meals. Use lean beef, cook it without fat and bulk out the mash with leeks to reduce the calories.*

Place a large non-stick saucepan or flameproof casserole dish over a medium heat. Add the mince and cook it with the onions, celery and carrots for 10 minutes until lightly coloured. Use a couple of wooden spoons to break up the meat as it cooks.

Stir in the tomatoes, tomato purée, beef stock, Worcestershire sauce and mixed herbs. Season with a good pinch of salt and plenty of freshly ground black pepper. Bring to the boil, then reduce the heat, cover loosely and simmer gently for 40 minutes, stirring occasionally until the mince is tender.

About 20 minutes before the meat is ready, make the potato topping. Peel the potatoes and cut them into rough 4cm chunks. Put them in a large saucepan and cover with cold water. Bring to the boil, then turn down the heat slightly and simmer for 18–20 minutes or until the potatoes are very tender. Heat the oil in a non-stick frying pan and fry the leeks for 5 minutes until softened but not coloured, stirring often. Drain the potatoes, then tip them back into the pan, season to taste and mash with the crème fraiche until smooth. Stir in the sautéed leeks and set aside.

Preheat the oven to 220°C/Fan 200°C/Gas 7. When the beef has been simmering for 40 minutes, mix the cornflour with the cold water to make a smooth paste. Stir this into the beef and cook for another 1–2 minutes or until the sauce is thickened, stirring often.

Pour the beef mixture into a 2-litre shallow ovenproof dish. Using a large spoon, top the beef with the mashed potatoes and leeks. Spoon the mixture all around the edge of the dish before heading into the middle, then fluff up with a fork.

Bake for 30 minutes until the topping is golden and the filling is bubbling. If making this ahead of time, let the pie cool, then cover and put in the fridge. Cook from chilled in a preheated oven at 210°C/Fan 190°/Gas 6½ for 40–50 minutes or until the pie is piping hot throughout.

**SERVES 6–8**

400g lean minced beef
2 medium onions, chopped
2 celery sticks, finely sliced
2 medium carrots, diced
400g can of chopped tomatoes
2 tbsp tomato purée
500ml beef stock, made with 1 beef stock cube
1 tbsp Worcestershire sauce
1 tsp dried mixed herbs
4 tsp cornflour
1 tbsp cold water
flaked sea salt
freshly ground black pepper

**Leeky potato topping**
750g floury potatoes, such as King Edwards or Maris Pipers
2 tsp sunflower oil
2 slender leeks, trimmed and cut into 1cm slices
150g half-fat crème fraiche
flaked sea salt
freshly ground black pepper

---

*322 calories per portion (if serving 6)*
*242 calories per portion (if serving 8)*

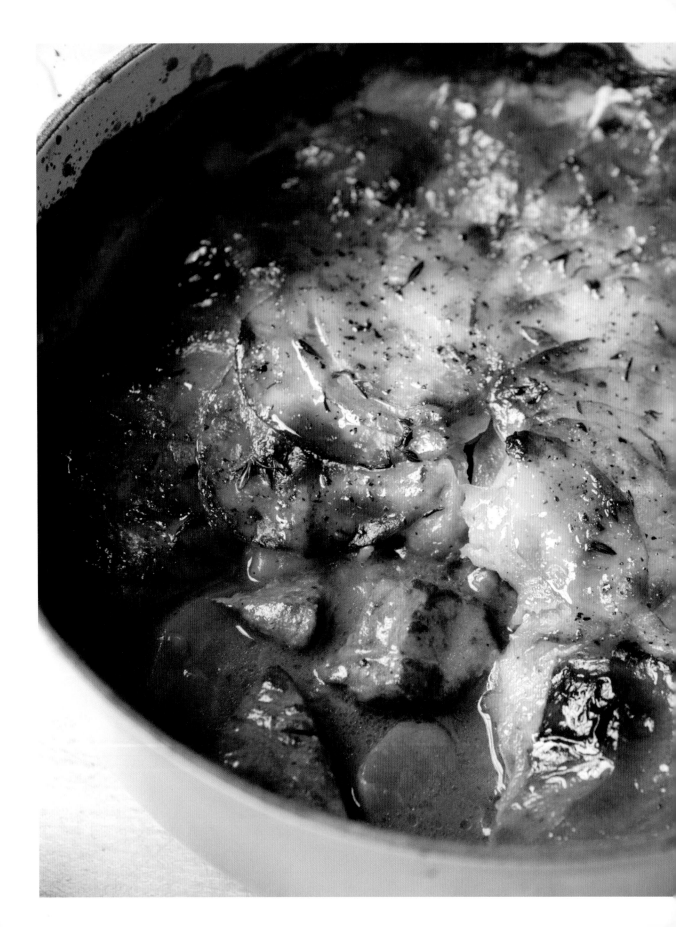

# LEAN LAMB HOTPOT

*We've always loved this simple old-fashioned dish and this is our new-wave version – who'd have thought it? By trimming the meat well and reducing the amount of potatoes, we've made this lower in calories than the trad recipe. Makes a cracking supper on a cold day, served with lots of green veg.*

Trim any visible fat off the lamb and cut the meat into rough 3cm chunks. Season generously all over with salt and pepper.

Heat the oil in a large non-stick frying pan and fry the lamb in 2 batches over a medium-high heat until nicely browned on all sides. Transfer the browned meat to a medium casserole dish– it will need to hold about 2.5 litres.

Tip the onions and carrots into the pan with the lamb and sprinkle with the flour. Toss everything together well, then pour over the stock and add the thyme leaves, rosemary and Worcestershire sauce. Stir well.

Preheat the oven to 170°C/Fan 150°C/Gas 3½. Peel the potatoes and cut them into slices about 5mm thick. Arrange the slices on top of the lamb, overlapping and layering them as you go. Season with ground black pepper and cover with a tight-fitting lid.

Bake the hotpot for 1 hour, then remove the lid and bake for a further 45 minutes or until the potatoes are nicely browned and the lamb is tender. Check by poking with the point of a knife into the centre of the lamb filling – if the meat is done the knife should slide in easily. Serve with freshly cooked greens.

**SERVES 4**

700g well-trimmed lamb leg meat (or leg steaks)
2 tsp sunflower oil
2 medium onions, peeled and thinly sliced
5 medium carrots, peeled and thickly sliced (about 300g prepared weight)
3 tbsp plain flour
600ml lamb stock, made with 1 lamb stock cube
1 tbsp fresh thyme leaves or ½ tsp dried thyme
1 rosemary stalk or ½ tsp dried rosemary
2 tbsp Worcestershire sauce
flaked sea salt
freshly ground black pepper

**Potato topping**
3 medium potatoes (about 500g)

*438 calories per portion*

# SI AND DAVE'S WEIGHT-LOSS TIPS

———

Stews taste rich and luxurious – the very opposite of what you think of as diet food – but we've found that they don't have to be high in calories.

———

When making stews, lightly brown the meat in a very small amount of oil. There's no need to use a lot.

———

Add vegetables and pulses to your stews. They all help to fill you up without too many calories.

———

Spice is good. A spicy stew is full of flavour and we think it helps you feel more satisfied.

———

Cook just a 50g portion of rice or pasta to have with some of the lower-calorie stews. If you fill the rest of your plate with lots of colourful vegetables or salad, you will hardly notice. And you have the extra treat of all those nutritious, fibre-rich vegetables to munch through – so you'll feel full and virtuous at the same time.

———

Stews are great family meals and are easy to prepare ahead. Serve with extra carbs for the kids or skinny family members.

———

# STEWS

"Small changes in cooking
habits can make a big
difference to your waistline."

*Dave*

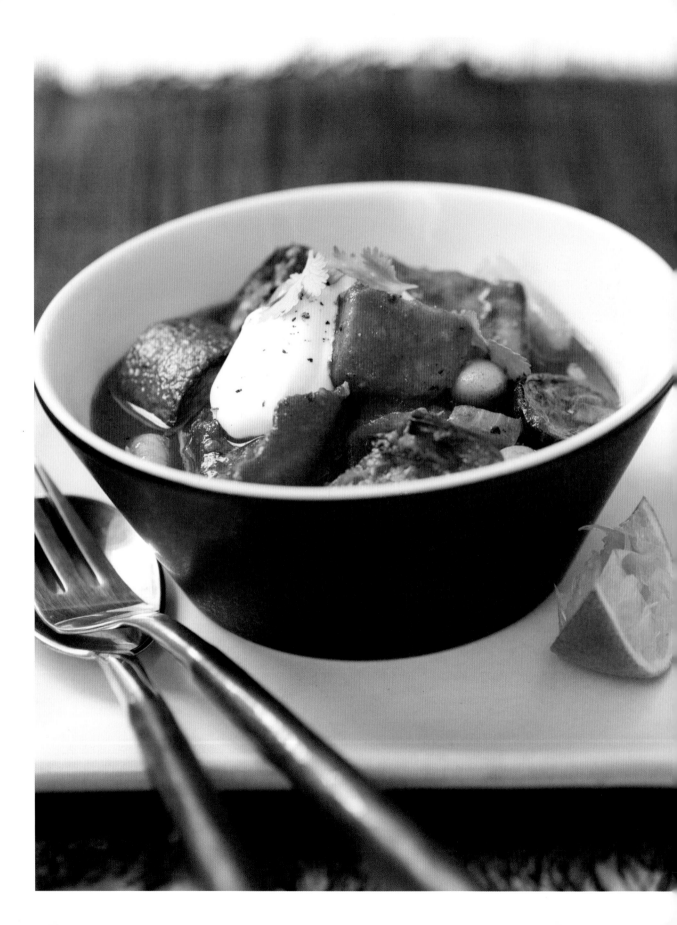

# SPICY BEAN AND VEGETABLE STEW

*This is a really substantial, flavoursome stew that will please veggies and non-veggies alike. By leaving out meat, you can enjoy hearty portions of pulses and vegetables while staying within a sensible calorie count.*

Heat the oil in a large, deep non-stick frying pan, saucepan or sauté pan. Stir-fry the aubergine over a high heat for 3 minutes until nicely browned. Add the onions to the pan and cook for 2 minutes, stirring often. Scatter the peppers and sweet potato into the pan and stir-fry with the aubergine and onions for another 4 minutes. Sprinkle over the spices and cook for 1 minute, stirring constantly.

Add the chopped tomatoes and beans and stir in the 600ml of water. Season with a good pinch of salt, bring to a simmer and cook for 10 minutes, stirring occasionally. Add the courgette, return to a simmer and cook for a further 10 minutes, stirring regularly.

Mix the cornflour with the 2 teaspoons of water to make a thin paste and stir this into the bean mixture. Cook for 5 minutes or until the sweet potato is just tender and the sauce is thick. Stir regularly, especially towards the end of the cooking time to prevent the sauce sticking. If it does start to stick, add a splash of water.

Remove the pan from the heat, stir in the lime juice and serve the stew topped with half-fat crème fraiche and scattered with fresh coriander leaves if you like. Add lime wedges for squeezing.

**SERVES 4–5**

1 tbsp olive oil
1 small aubergine (about 250g), cut into 3cm dice
2 medium onions, halved and finely sliced
1 yellow pepper, deseeded and cut into 3cm dice
1 red pepper, deseeded and cut into 3cm dice
1 medium sweet potato (300g), peeled and cut into 2cm dice
1 tsp ground coriander
½–1 tsp hot chilli powder
½ tsp smoked paprika (hot)
400g can of chopped tomatoes
400g can of cannellini beans, rinsed and drained
600ml cold water
1 large courgette, halved lengthways and cut into 1.5cm slices
2 tsp cornflour
2 tsp cold water
freshly squeezed juice of ½ lime
4 tbsp half-fat crème fraiche
flaked sea salt
fresh coriander leaves, to garnish (optional)
lime wedges, for squeezing

*299 calories per portion (if serving 4)*
*239 calories per portion (if serving 5)*

# GORGEOUS FISH STEW
# WITH GARLIC CROUTONS

*Light in calories but heavy on flavour, our fish stew is a real treat for foodies. You don't have to add the topping but it makes the meal even more special – great if you've got friends coming round. Add some fresh mussels to the stew at the same time as the cod if you like.*

**SERVES 4**

1 tbsp olive oil
1 medium onion, finely sliced
2 celery sticks, very finely sliced
2 large garlic cloves, peeled and finely sliced
250g potatoes, preferably Maris Pipers
1 yellow pepper
2 tsp ground coriander
good pinch of saffron threads
2 bay leaves
150ml white wine
400g can of chopped tomatoes
1 heaped tbsp tomato purée
600ml cold water
½ fish stock cube
2 tsp caster sugar
½ tsp flaked sea salt, plus extra for seasoning
150g fine green beans
400g thick white fish fillet
200g cooked and peeled king prawns, thawed
freshly ground black pepper
freshly chopped flat-leaf parsley

**Topping**

4 long, thin diagonal slices of ciabatta bread (each about 20g)
2 tbsp light mayonnaise
1 garlic clove, peeled and crushed
15g Parmesan cheese, finely grated

---

*289 calories per portion*
*(without ciabatta)*
*366 calories per portion (with ciabatta)*

Heat the oil in a large flameproof casserole dish or wide, heavy-based saucepan and gently fry the onion and celery for 8 minutes until well softened, stirring occasionally. Add the garlic and cook for 2 minutes more. Don't let the garlic burn or it will give your stew a bitter flavour. If the onion starts to stick, add a splash of cold water to the pan. Meanwhile, peel the potatoes and cut them into rough 2cm chunks. Deseed the pepper and cut that into chunks too.

Stir the ground coriander, saffron and bay leaves into the casserole and cook for another couple of minutes, stirring constantly. Pour over the wine and let it all bubble for a few seconds before adding the yellow pepper, potatoes, chopped tomatoes, tomato purée, water, stock cube and sugar. Season with the ½ teaspoon of salt and plenty of ground black pepper.

Bring the stew to a gentle simmer and cook uncovered for 15 minutes, stirring occasionally, until the potatoes are softened but not breaking apart. Trim the green beans, cut them in half and add them to the pan, then return to a simmer. Cook for a further 5 minutes, stirring occasionally. Season with more salt and pepper to taste.

Remove the skin from the fish fillets and cut the fish into rough 2.5cm chunks. Drop the fish pieces on top of the bubbling liquid and cover the pan with a lid. Poach the fish over a medium heat for 3 minutes or until it is almost cooked. Remove the lid and very gently stir in the prawns, trying not to break up the fish too much. Cover again and simmer for 2 minutes more or until the fish is opaque and the prawns are hot. Don't let the prawns overcook.

While the fish is simmering, toast or griddle the ciabatta bread and mix the mayonnaise with the garlic. Ladle the stew into warmed deep plates or bowls. Scatter with roughly chopped flat-leaf parsley. Spread the hot toast with the garlic mayonnaise and place on top of each bowl or serve on the side. Sprinkle with grated Parmesan and serve.

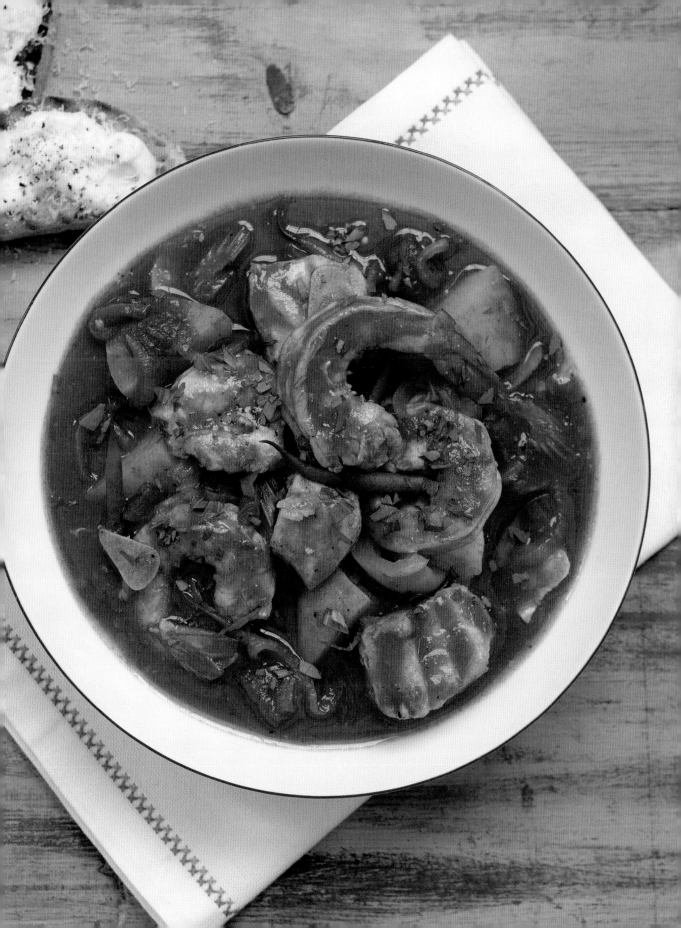

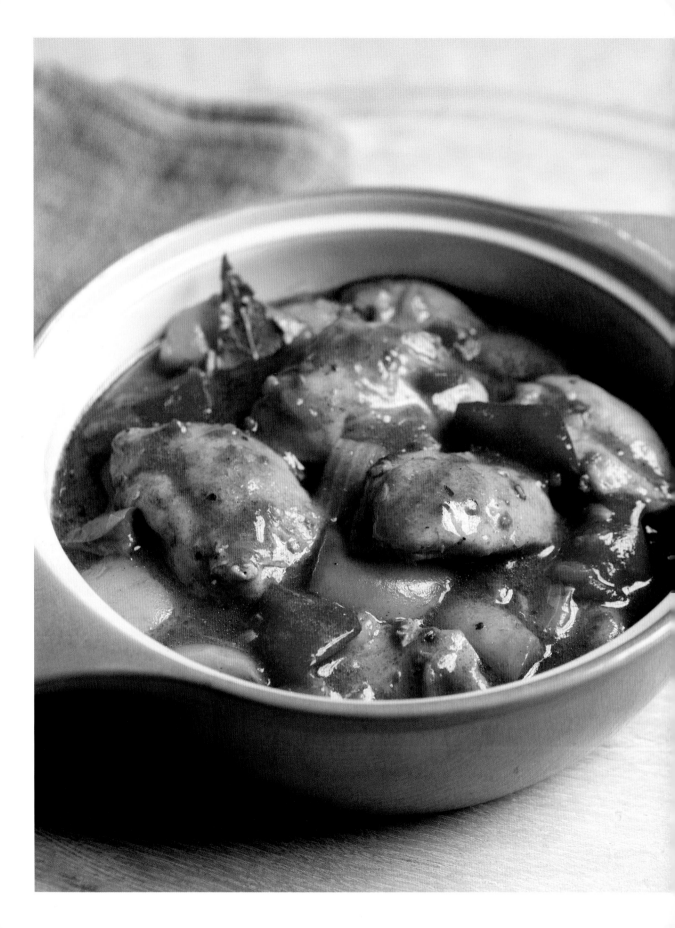

# PAPRIKA CHICKEN

*This is a low-cal version of a popular Romanian dish called paprikash, which we both love. By making a few little changes, like skinning the chicken, we can still enjoy this excellent feast while on a diet. Just brilliant.*

Heat the oil in a large non-stick saucepan or casserole dish and fry the onions over a medium heat for 6–8 minutes until softened and lightly coloured, stirring regularly. Put the chicken on a board and cut away any visible fat. Cut each thigh in half, season with ground black pepper and add to the pan.

Cook the chicken with the onions for 4–5 minutes until lightly coloured on each side. Stir in the garlic and paprika and cook for 1 minute more. Tip the tomatoes into the pan, pour over the chicken stock and add the bay leaves and mixed herbs. Bring to a gentle simmer, then cover the pan loosely with a lid and cook for 20 minutes, stirring occasionally.

While the vegetables are cooking, cut the peppers in half and deseed. Cut them into chunky pieces, each about 3cm. Add the peppers to the chicken and cook everything for another 25–35 minutes, stirring occasionally, until the chicken is tender.

Mix the cornflour and water together to make a smooth paste and stir this into the pan. Cook for 2–3 minutes until the sauce is thickened, stirring constantly.

Serve the paprika chicken topped with a little half-fat crème fraiche. Lovely with a small portion of rice or some mashed potatoes.

**SERVES 6**

1 tbsp sunflower oil

2 medium onions, halved and finely sliced

12 boneless, skinless chicken thighs

2 garlic cloves, peeled and crushed

1 tbsp smoked paprika (or plain paprika if you prefer)

400g can of chopped tomatoes

400ml chicken stock (fresh or made with 1 stock cube)

2 bay leaves

1 tsp dried mixed herbs

3 large peppers, red, yellow and green

1 tbsp cornflour

1 tbsp cold water

6 tbsp half-fat crème fraiche

freshly ground black pepper

*282 calories per portion*

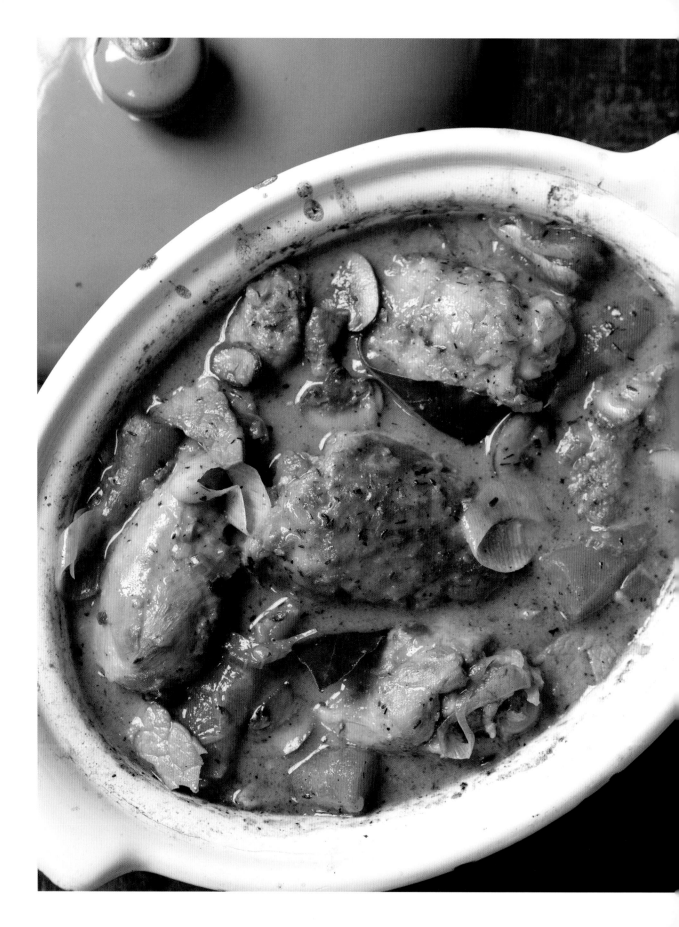

# OLD-FASHIONED CHICKEN AND VEGETABLE STEW

*The cider and bacon add a touch of sweetness and extra flavour to the chicken and veg, making this a lovely supper dish. Keep it low-fat by removing the skin from the chicken legs before cooking and using as little oil as possible for browning the meat and vegetables.*

Mix the flour and thyme with a good pinch of salt and plenty of freshly ground black pepper in a large strong freezer bag. Strip the skin off the chicken legs and put them on a board. Break the joint of each leg by bending it in the opposite direction. You may hear a small crack. Cut each leg quarter in half with a sturdy knife to give 8 chicken portions. Using a good set of kitchen scissors, trim off any visible fat.

Put the chicken portions in the freezer bag, a few at a time, and shake well until they are evenly coated in the flour. Heat the oil in a large non-stick frying pan over a medium heat and fry the chicken, a few pieces at a time, until golden brown all over. As they are browned, transfer the chicken pieces to a large flameproof casserole dish. Preheat the oven to 180°C/Fan 160°C/Gas 4.

Put the bacon, onions and celery in the pan used for browning the chicken and fry for 4–5 minutes over medium heat until lightly browned, stirring often. Add the mushrooms and cook for 2 minutes more, then tip everything into the casserole dish with the chicken pieces. Sprinkle in any flour remaining in the freezer bag and stir well.

Pour about half the cider into the frying pan and stir vigorously with a wooden spoon to lift any sediment from the bottom. Simmer for a few seconds, then pour into the casserole. Add the rest of the cider and the stock, then stir in the carrots and bay leaves and bring to a simmer on the hob.

Cover with a lid and cook in the centre of the oven for 1 hour, then remove the casserole from the oven and stir in the leeks. Pop the dish back into the oven for a further 30–40 minutes or until the chicken is tender and the sauce thickened. Serve with some green beans or spring greens.

**SERVES 4**

3 tbsp plain flour
2 tsp dried thyme
4 chicken leg quarters
2 tbsp sunflower oil
4 rashers of rindless smoked back bacon, cut into 1cm-wide strips
2 medium onions, chopped
2 celery sticks, thinly sliced
150g small chestnut mushrooms, wiped and sliced or quartered if large
500ml bottle of dry cider
300ml chicken stock, made with 1 chicken stock cube
2 bay leaves
400g Chantenay or other small fat carrots, trimmed and peeled
2 slender leeks, trimmed and cut into 2cm slices
flaked sea salt
freshly ground black pepper

*435 calories per portion*

# OUR SPECIAL CASSOULET

*Cassoulet is a hearty dish but with a few little tweaks we've reduced the calorie count while keeping the big flavours. Choose really meaty sausages and gammon, take the skin off the chicken and use a very small amount of oil – it all helps. We kept a rugby team happy with this!*

**SERVES 6**

½ tsp sunflower oil
6 good-quality herby sausages, at least 85% meat
4 celery sticks
3 medium carrots
2 medium onions, halved and sliced
6 boneless, skinless chicken thighs (about 450g)
2 fat garlic cloves, crushed
200g piece of smoked lean gammon, trimmed and cut into 2cm cubes
2 x 400g cans of chopped tomatoes
150ml red wine (or water)
300ml cold water
1 tsp caster sugar
1 tsp dried chilli flakes
1 bay leaf
4–5 bushy sprigs of fresh thyme
400g can of cannellini beans in water, drained and rinsed
400g can of butter beans in water, drained and rinsed
freshly ground black pepper

**Garnish**
handful of fresh flat-leaf parsley
finely grated zest of ½ well-scrubbed large orange

Brush a large non-stick frying pan with the sunflower oil, using the tip of a pastry brush. Add the sausages to the pan and cook over a medium heat for 10 minutes, turning every now and then until nicely browned on all sides. Meanwhile, trim the celery and peel the carrots and cut them into diagonal slices about 1.5 centimetres thick.

Preheat the oven to 180°C/Fan 160°C/Gas 4. Add the onions to the frying pan and cook with the sausages for 6–8 minutes, stirring regularly until softened and lightly browned.

Trim the chicken thighs of any visible fat – we find a good pair of kitchen scissors does the job well – then cut them in half. Add the garlic and chicken pieces to the pan with the sausages and onions and cook for 3–4 minutes, turning the chicken twice until coloured all over. Transfer everything to a large flameproof casserole dish.

Stir in the gammon, celery, carrots, tomatoes, red wine and water, then sprinkle over the caster sugar and chilli flakes. Stir in the bay leaf and thyme and season with lots of ground black pepper. Bring to a simmer on the hob, then cover with a lid and transfer to the oven. Cook for 45 minutes.

Take the casserole out of the oven and stir in all the beans. Cover with the lid again and put the dish back in the oven for another 30 minutes.

Just before the cassoulet is ready, prepare the garnish. Chop the parsley roughly and toss with the orange zest in a serving dish. Serve large portions of the cassoulet in deep plates or wide bowls with a good sprinkling of the zesty parsley garnish on each one.

*464 calories per portion*

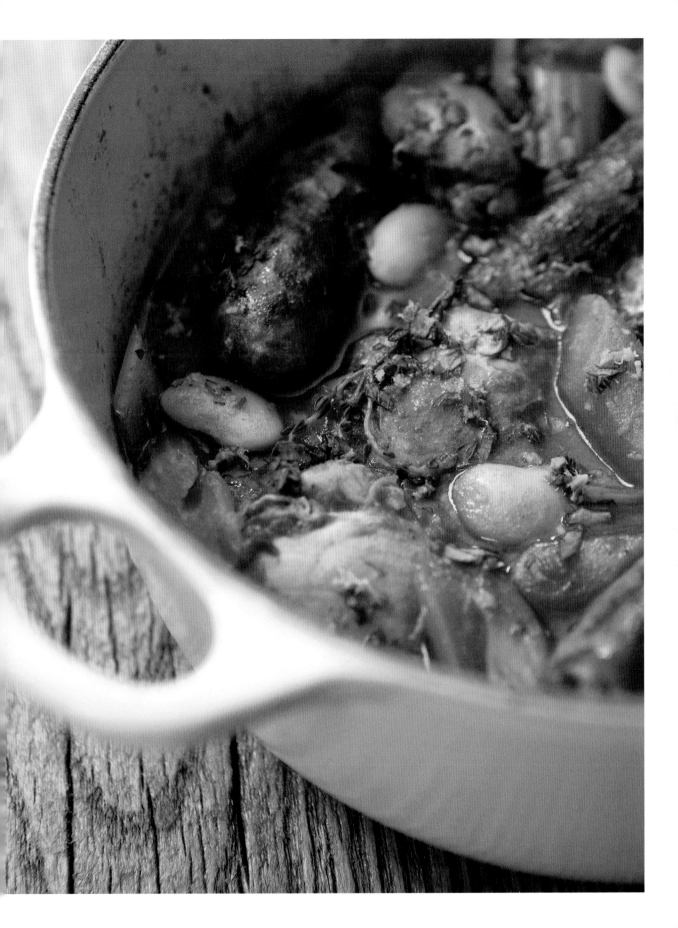

# RICH BEEF AND ALE CASSEROLE

*We do love a good stew and we've discovered that you don't need to brown the meat in loads of fat. In this recipe we use lean meat and only a tablespoon of oil and the stew still tastes really rich and satisfying. Serve with some light mash that you soften with half-fat crème fraiche and bulk out with some steamed leeks for a cracking good feast.*

**SERVES 6**

1 tbsp sunflower oil
2 medium onions, chopped
4 tbsp plain flour
1 tsp flaked sea salt
2 tsp dried mixed herbs
1kg lean braising beef
1 bay leaf
500ml dark ale or stout
250ml beef stock, made with
1 beef stock cube
2 tbsp tomato purée
2 tsp caster sugar
5 medium carrots (about 275g),
peeled and thickly sliced
2 parsnips (about 300g), peeled,
halved lengthways and sliced
freshly ground black pepper

*377 calories per portion
(without the mash)*

Preheat the oven to 180°C/Fan 160°C/Gas 4. Heat the oil in a large flameproof casserole dish. Add the onions and fry them over a medium-high heat for about 5 minutes until lightly browned, stirring regularly. Remove the pan from the heat.

Put the flour, salt and dried herbs in a large bowl and season with lots of freshly ground black pepper. Trim the beef of any hard fat and sinew, then cut the meat into rough 3cm cubes. Toss the meat in the flour until evenly coated, then tip it into the casserole dish with the onions.

Add the bay leaf, ale, stock, tomato purée and sugar. Stir well and bring to the boil, then cover with a lid. Carefully transfer the casserole to the oven and cook for 1½ hours. At the end of this time, take the casserole out of the oven and stir in the carrots and parsnips. Put the lid back on and return the dish to the oven for a further 45 minutes or until the beef and vegetables are tender.

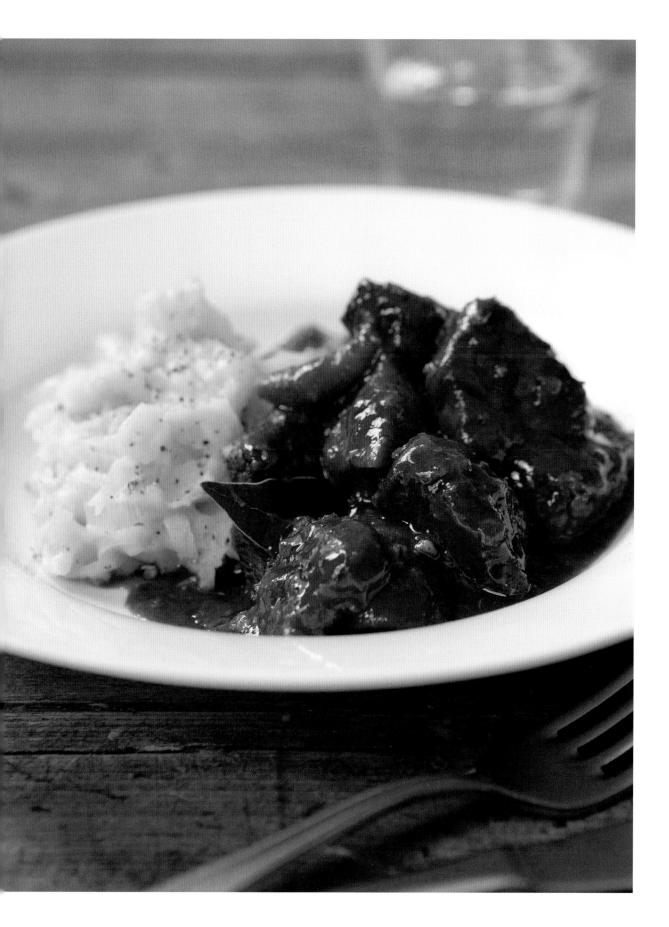

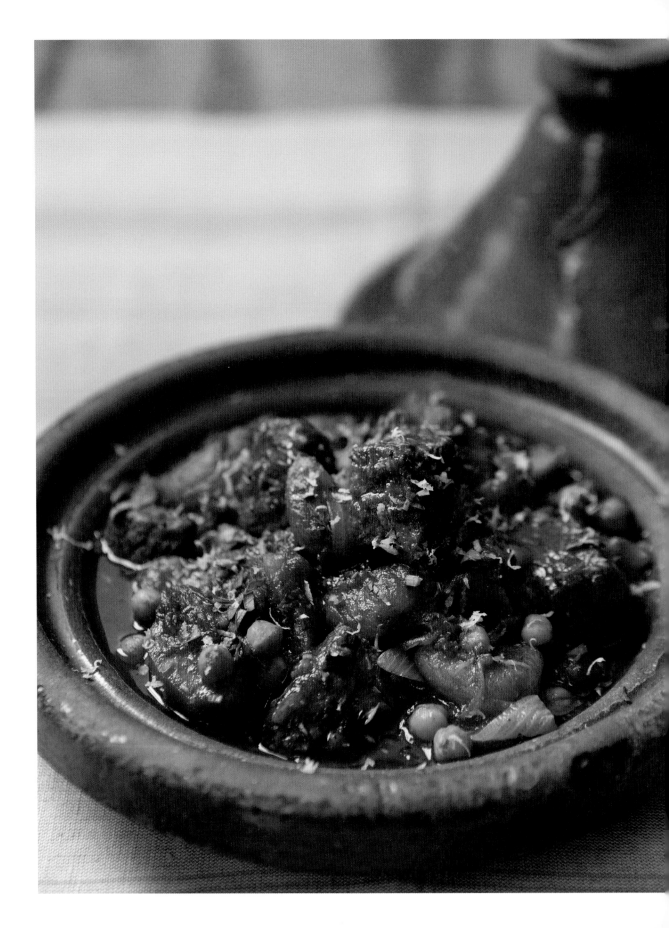

# LAMB TAGINE

*A tagine is a kind of spicy stew which originates from Morocco. This is our special version that is made with lean meat and less oil than usual but still tastes the business. Serve with a lightly dressed salad or some gorgeous green beans.*

Preheat the oven to 180°C/Fan 160°C/Gas 4. Trim the lamb of any hard fat and cut the meat into rough 3cm chunks. Season all over with salt and pepper. Mix the cumin, coriander, cinnamon and chilli powder in a small bowl.

Heat the oil in a large flameproof casserole dish or saucepan. Add the lamb, onions and garlic and stir-fry over a high heat for 1 minute until lightly coloured. Sprinkle with the spices and cook for 1–2 minutes more, tossing constantly. Take the pan off the heat as soon as the spices begin to give off a strong aroma.

Tip the tomatoes into the casserole dish and add the water, honey and chickpeas. Crumble the stock cube over the top and stir well. Bring to a simmer on the hob, stirring a couple of times, then cover the dish with a lid and put it in the preheated oven. Cook for 1 hour.

Just before the lamb is due to come out of the oven, peel the sweet potato and cut it into rough 2.5cm chunks. Carefully remove the casserole from the oven and stir in the sweet potato and apricots. Put the lid back on and return the casserole to the oven. Cook for another 45–60 minutes or until the lamb is very tender.

Serve the tagine sprinkled with some roughly chopped flat-leaf parsley tossed with a little very finely grated lemon zest if you like. The zest adds a little extra spark of flavour.

**SERVES 5**

750g lean lamb leg meat
(or leg steaks)
2 tsp ground cumin
2 tsp ground coriander
½ tsp ground cinnamon
1 tsp hot chilli powder
1 tbsp sunflower oil
2 medium onions, halved and sliced
2 garlic cloves, peeled and
finely chopped
400g can of chopped tomatoes
500ml cold water
3 tbsp runny honey
400g can of chickpeas, drained
and rinsed
1 lamb stock cube
1 medium sweet potato (about
250g)
75g no-soak dried apricots, halved
flaked sea salt
freshly ground black pepper
fresh flat-leaf parsley and finely
grated lemon zest, to serve
(optional)

*457 calories per portion*

# SI AND DAVE'S WEIGHT-LOSS TIPS

———

Try to keep starchy carbohydrate portions down – a couple of
new potatoes or a small baked potato should be plenty while you
are trying to lose weight. Or serve green vegetables which are much
lower in calories, and juicy veg such as courgettes and peppers.

———

If you do want some carbs, choose vegetables such as squash and
carrots, which are lower in calories than potatoes. Beetroot
is great too – really meaty and full of goodness.

———

Mega salads take a while to eat so help you feel satisfied.
Add protein such as chicken strips or tuna to salads, as it makes
them more filling. Look for tuna packed in water, not oil,
to reduce the calorie count.

———

When you've piled your plate high with salad, don't slather it with
high-cal dressing. Low-cal bought dressings are fine or try making
your own with the recipes in this book (see page 111).
Keep the fat content as low as possible.

———

Be under no illusions – despite its healthy image olive oil has as
many calories as butter. It may be better for you but the effect on
your weight is the same.

———

# VEGETABLES & SALADS

"Some food groups are more forgiving than others. Just like your mum always said, you can eat lots more veg than bread and potatoes."

*Si*

# POSH PRAWN COCKTAIL

*The traditional prawn cocktail gets its high calorie count from the dressing, not the ingredients, but there's nothing to fear in this version. We've substantially cut the calories in the dressing while not compromising on flavour. Get your laughing gear round this and enjoy.*

**SERVES 4**

50g light mayonnaise
2 tsp tomato ketchup
½ tsp Worcestershire sauce
¼ tsp celery salt (optional)
200g cooked and peeled king
prawns, thawed and drained
2 baby gem lettuces, leaves separated
12 cherry tomatoes
¼ cucumber, sliced
100g smoked salmon, cut into
wide strips
½ tsp paprika
freshly ground black pepper
lemon wedges, for squeezing

*139 calories per portion*

Mix the mayonnaise, ketchup, Worcestershire sauce, celery salt (if using) and lots of freshly ground black pepper in a bowl. Stir in the prawns. Arrange the lettuce leaves in wide glass dessert dishes or shred the leaves and pile into stemmed wine glasses.

Arrange the tomatoes and cucumber on top of the lettuce, then spoon in the prawn cocktail mixture. Arrange strips of smoked salmon on the prawns, then sprinkle with a little paprika and some ground black pepper. Add lemon wedges for squeezing and serve.

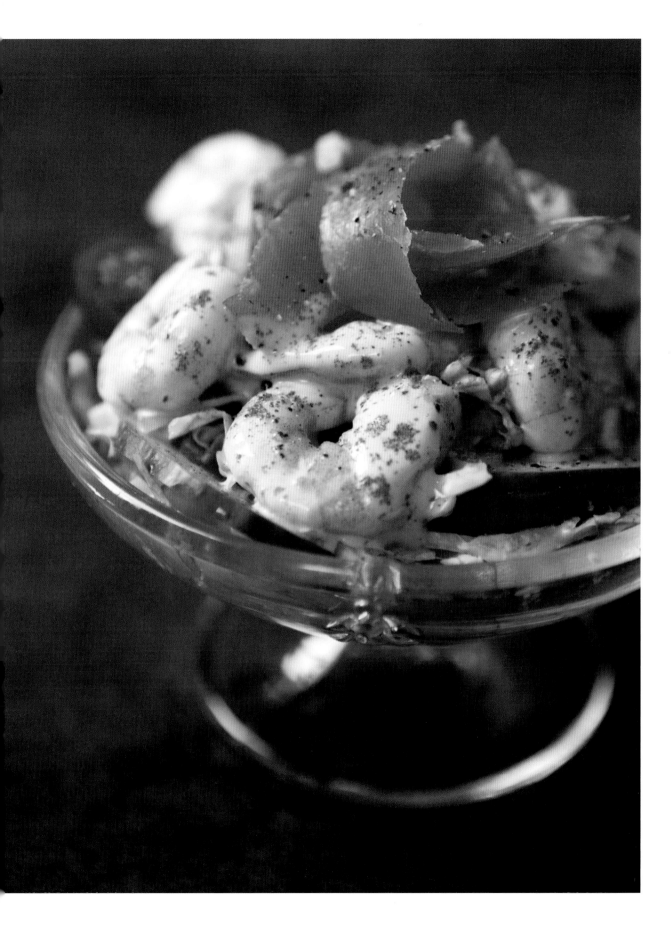

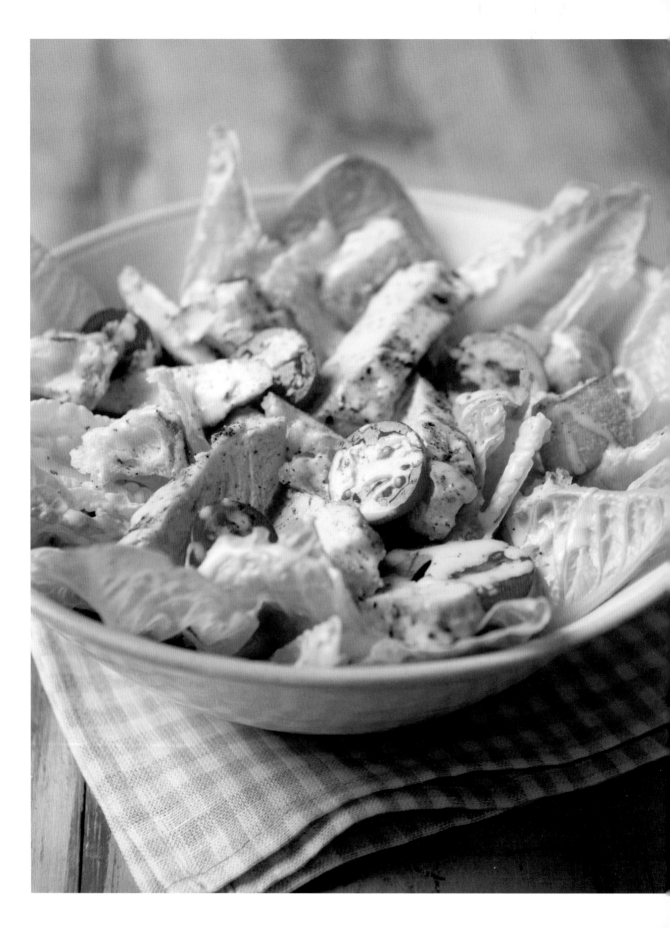

# CHICKEN CAESAR SALAD

*We've been creating and enjoying loads of salads and we love this one which is good and hearty. The clever little dressing makes enough for four servings, so cover what's left and keep it in the fridge for up to three days. Use it to perk up any salad leaves.*

To make the dressing, put the anchovy fillets in a pestle and mortar, add the chopped garlic clove and pound into a paste. Add the mayonnaise, lemon juice, Parmesan and water and stir well to make a pourable dressing.

Place a chicken breast between 2 sheets of cling film and bash it with a rolling pin until the chicken is about 1cm thick. Bash the other chicken breast in the same way, then season the breasts on both sides with a little salt and plenty of black pepper.

Dip a pastry brush in the oil and brush over the base of a large non-stick frying pan. Place the pan over a medium heat, add the chicken and cook for 2 minutes. Turn the breasts over and cook for 2–3 minutes on the other side until nicely browned and cooked through. Remove from the heat and leave the chicken in the warm pan to rest.

While the chicken is cooking, make the salad. Separate the lettuce leaves and wash and drain them well. Tear any large leaves into smaller pieces. Arrange the lettuce in a large serving dish and scatter over the tomatoes. Toast the slices of ciabatta and tear them into bite-sized pieces.

Put the cooked chicken breasts on a board and cut them into thick strips. Scatter these over the lettuce and tomatoes and toss everything together lightly. Spoon over half the dressing and serve while the chicken is warm. Fantastic!

**SERVES 2**

2 boneless, skinless chicken breasts
1 tsp sunflower oil
1 romaine lettuce heart
10 cherry tomatoes, halved
2 slices of ciabatta bread, each about
1.5cm thick (15g a slice)
flaked sea salt
freshly ground black pepper

**Dressing**

2 anchovy fillets in oil, drained and
roughly chopped
1 garlic clove, peeled and
roughly chopped
2 tbsp light mayonnaise
1 tsp lemon juice
15g Parmesan cheese, finely grated
2½ tbsp cold water

*272 calories per portion*

# CHILLI SALAD BOWLS

*This is one of the gutsiest salads we've come up with – packed with beef and flavour. A proper Hairy Dieters' feast. If you like, you can also make this with ready-made taco shells which are even lower in calories than tortillas so you can eat more filling!*

**SERVES 4**

300g lean minced beef (less than 10% fat)
1 small onion, finely chopped
2 garlic cloves, peeled and crushed
1 tsp ground cumin
1 tsp ground coriander
1 tsp hot chilli powder
2 tbsp tomato purée
½ tsp caster sugar
300ml beef stock, made with 1 beef stock cube
4 large flour tortillas
1 tsp sunflower oil
1 romaine lettuce or 3 baby gem lettuces, leaves thickly shredded
3 ripe vine tomatoes, sliced
15cm piece of cucumber, sliced
4 spring onions, trimmed and sliced
freshly squeezed juice of ½ lime
40g mature Cheddar cheese
4 tbsp half-fat crème fraiche
4 tbsp fresh tomato salsa sauce
flaked sea salt
freshly ground black pepper

*397 calories per portion*

Put the minced beef, onion and garlic in a medium non-stick saucepan and cook over a high heat for 5 minutes, stirring with 2 wooden spoons to break up any clumps of meat. Stir in the cumin, coriander and chilli and cook for 2 minutes more, stirring constantly.

Add the tomato purée, sugar and beef stock and bring to a simmer. Cover the pan and leave to simmer gently over a low heat for 30 minutes. Remove the lid and stir the chilli mixture occasionally.

While the beef is cooking, prepare the tortilla bowls. Preheat the oven to 200°C/Fan 180°C/Gas 6. Take a sheet of foil about 1 metre long and scrunch it up into a ball about 10cm in diameter. Place it in the centre of a large baking sheet.

Take a tortilla and brush the centre on 1 side with a little of the oil – this will help prevent it sticking to the foil. Drape the tortilla over the ball of foil, oil-side down, pinching and loosely pleating it to create a bowl shape. Bake for 5 minutes until the bowl shape is set and the tortilla is lightly crisped.

Take the tortilla out of the oven and carefully remove it from the foil – it should be just cool enough to handle. Place the tortilla on an upturned tumbler and press to create a flat base on which to turn the tortilla once cold. The tortilla should still be warm enough to mould to the shape of the glass. Leave to cool while you make the next bowl in the same way. Put each upturned tortilla on a plate as soon as it is ready.

Remove the lid from the pan of beef and turn the heat up high. Cook for a further 4–5 minutes, stirring constantly, until most of the liquid has evaporated and the beef is looking fairly dry. Take the pan off the heat.

Toss the lettuce with the tomatoes, cucumber, spring onions and lime juice. Divide the salad between the tortilla bowls and season with black pepper, then top with the hot mince. Coarsely grate some Cheddar over each serving and add some crème fraiche and salsa. Tuck in while the beef is warm.

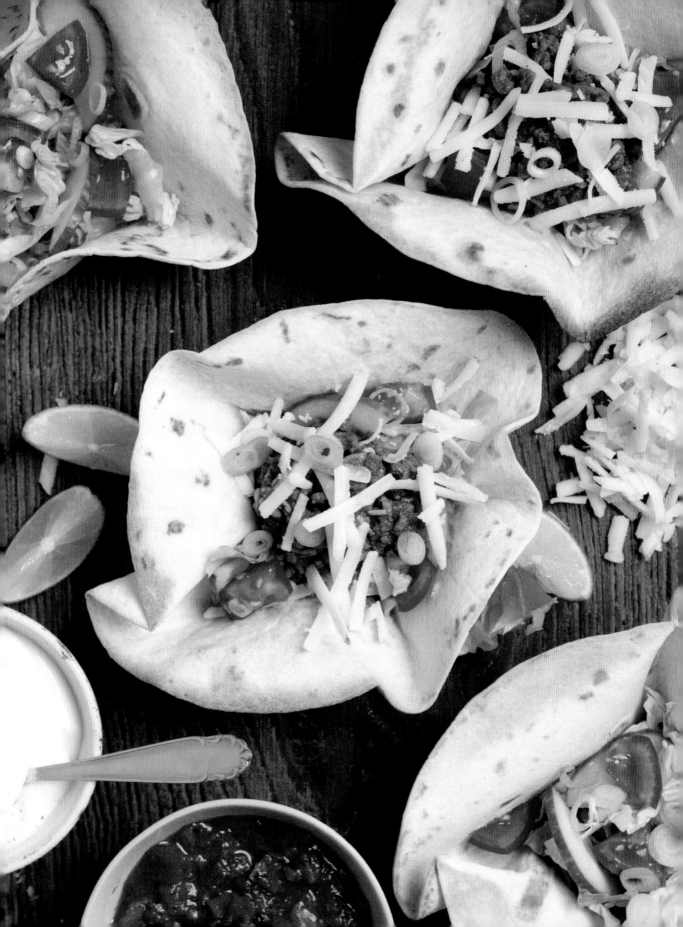

# CUMIN-CRUSTED VEGETABLES

*This is a lovely spicy variation on your classic roasties, using a small amount of oil and lots of tantalising tastes. Goes beautifully with our masala-marinated chicken, which you'll find on page 50, or with plain grilled meat.*

**SERVES 4–5**

600g medium potatoes, preferably
Maris Pipers
1 tsp black mustard seeds
1 tsp cumin seeds
2 tbsp sunflower oil
1 tsp garam masala
½ tsp turmeric
1 medium red onion, halved and
cut into thin wedges
1 yellow pepper, deseeded and cut
into 4cm chunks
1 red pepper, deseeded and cut into
4cm chunks
1 orange pepper, deseeded and cut
into 4cm chunks
2 medium courgettes, cut into
1cm slices
freshly ground black pepper

*199 calories per portion (if serving 4)*
*160 calories per portion (if serving 5)*

Preheat the oven to 210°C/Fan 190°C/Gas 6½. Half fill a medium saucepan with water and bring to the boil. Peel the potatoes, cut them into quarters and lower them carefully into the water. Bring the water back to the boil and cook for 5 minutes – just enough to parboil the spuds as though you're making them to go with your usual Sunday roast.

While the potatoes are boiling, place a large non-stick frying pan over a medium heat and add the mustard and cumin seeds. Toast for about 30 seconds, then stir in the oil, garam masala and turmeric. Sizzle for a few seconds and add the onion. Fry the onion in the spices for 1–2 minutes, stirring frequently.

Drain the potatoes in a large colander and toss several times to roughen up the surface of each potato. Tip them into the pan with the onion and spices, season with a few twists of ground black pepper and toss together until the potatoes are lightly coated. Tip everything on to a large baking tray and roast for 30 minutes.

Take the tray out of the oven and add the remaining vegetables. Toss lightly together and return to the oven for another 25–30 minutes until the potatoes are crisp and golden brown and the vegetables have softened.

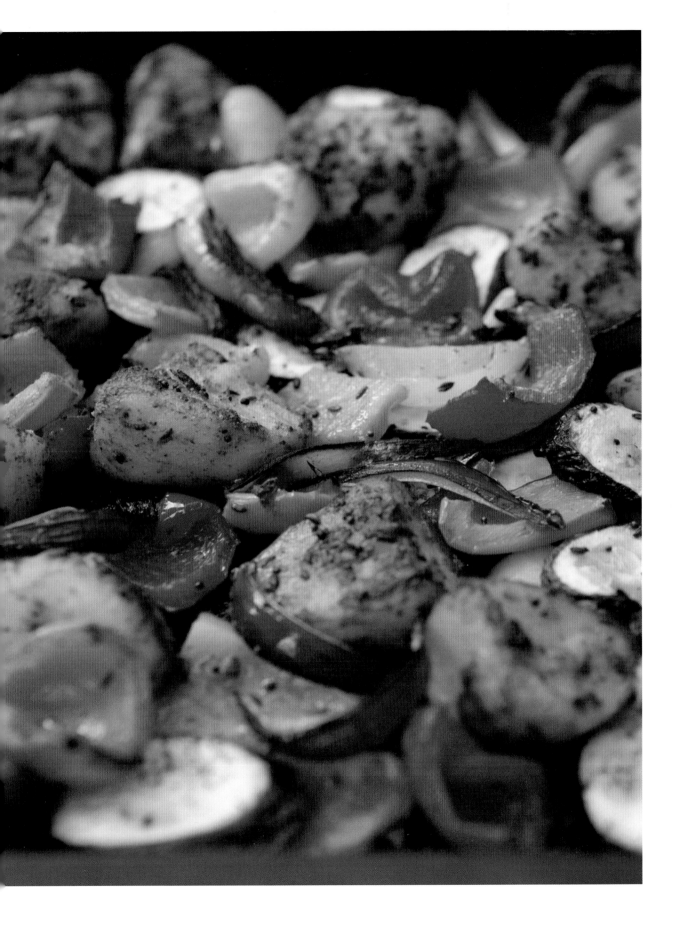

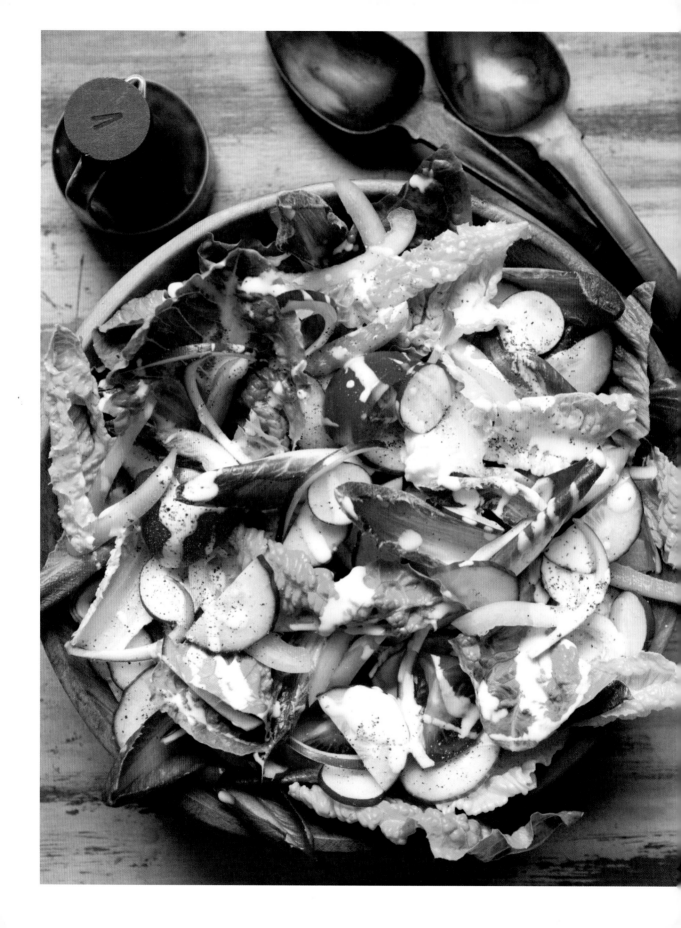

# GOOD BASIC MIXED SALAD

*A crisp mixed salad is a fantastic partner for so many dishes when you're watching your weight. It looks good, tastes good and takes a while to eat, which is always helpful when you're cutting down on calories and portions. Try some of our special dressings too.*

Separate the lettuce and chicory leaves and chuck away any that look wilted or damaged. Cut the larger chicory leaves in half lengthways. Rinse all the leaves in a colander under running water and drain well.

Cut the tomatoes into quarters and slice the radishes and cucumber, then cut the stalk off the pepper and scoop out and discard the seeds. Cut the pepper into rings or slices. Slice the onion or spring onions into very thin rings.

Scatter the leaves into a large serving bowl. Add the tomatoes and cucumber and toss lightly together, then scatter the radishes on top. Finish the salad with rings of pepper and red onion. Serve with one of the dressings below or a bought low-calorie dressing.

**SERVES 4–6**

1 romaine lettuce
1 chicory
3 ripe tomatoes
small handful of radishes
¼ cucumber
1 yellow pepper
½ red onion or 4 spring onions, trimmed

*44 calories per portion (if serving 4)*
*29 calories per portion (if serving 6)*

## VINAIGRETTE

Put 1 tablespoon of red wine vinegar, ½ crushed garlic clove, ¼ teaspoon of Dijon mustard, 1 teaspoon of caster sugar, a pinch of flaked sea salt and a couple of twists of black pepper in a small bowl and whisk with a metal balloon whisk until well combined. Gradually add 1 tablespoon extra virgin olive oil and whisk hard until the dressing thickens. Slowly whisk in 1 tablespoon of cold water. Adjust the seasoning to taste. **SERVES 6** *(20 calories per portion)*

## ZINGY YOGHURT DRESSING

Mix 4 tablespoons low-fat natural yoghurt, 2 teaspoons of freshly squeezed lemon juice and 1 teaspoon of runny honey in a small bowl until well combined. Stir in some finely chopped mint or coriander leaves if you like. **SERVES 6** *(8 calories per portion)*

## LIGHT HERBY DRESSING

Mix 3 tablespoons of light mayonnaise, ½ crushed garlic clove and a pinch of mixed dried herbs in a small bowl until well combined. Gradually add 3 tablespoons cold water, stirring well between each addition. Season with black pepper. **SERVES 6** *(22 calories per portion)*

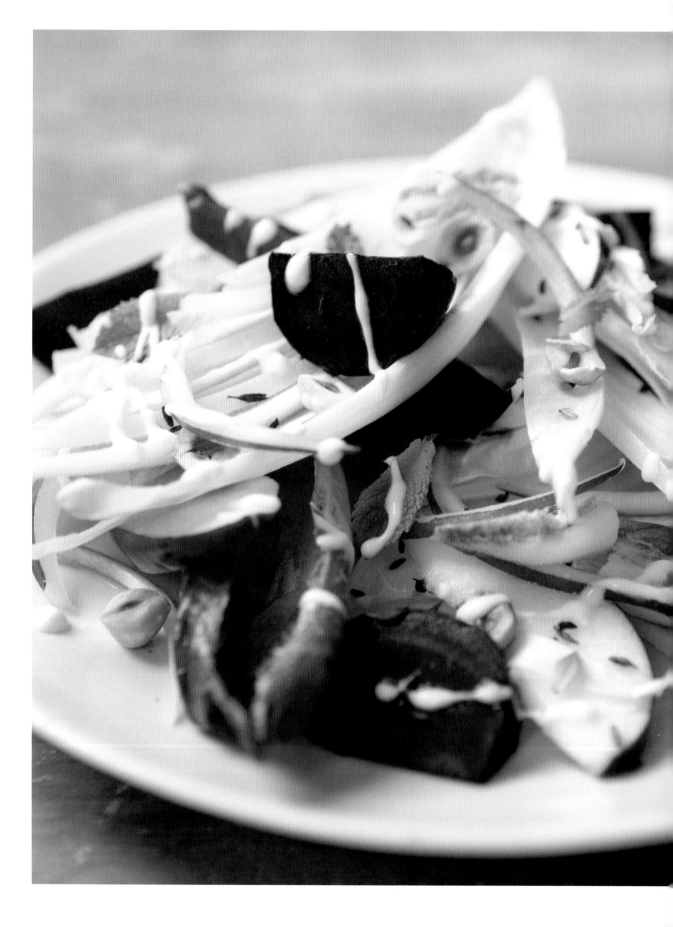

# BEETROOT SALAD WITH YOGHURT AND CUMIN SEEDS

*Beetroots are nutritious and have a lovely meaty texture. Cooked beets keep well in the fridge so cook a few to serve with other salads or warm with a little soft goat's cheese and snipped chives. They're good roasted too so if you have your oven on for another dish, wrap some beetroot in foil and cook at the same time. Ready-prepared beetroots are available in most supermarkets if you prefer – you'll need five or six of the baby ones for this dish. If you don't want purple fingers, wear clean rubber gloves when handling beetroots.*

Wash the beetroots well and trim off any stalks. Put them in a saucepan, cover with cold water and place over a high heat. Bring the water to the boil, then turn down the heat slightly, cover loosely with a lid and simmer for 50–60 minutes or until the beetroots are just tender. Check by testing them with the tip of a knife. Keep an eye on the water level and top up with extra water if necessary.

Drain the beetroots and leave them until cool enough to handle. Holding the beetroots under cold running water, gently slip off the skins, then cut them into wedges.

Roughly chop the hazelnuts on a board. Tip them into a colander and give it a good shake – all the tiny bits of nut should fall through the holes, leaving good chunky pieces for your salad.

Scatter the nuts into a non-stick frying pan and toast over a medium-high heat for 4–5 minutes or until lightly browned, turning them as they cook. Add the cumin seeds, if using, and toast together for 1–2 minutes, then set aside to cool. Mix the ingredients for the dressing in a small bowl.

Cut each head of chicory lengthways into 6 thin wedges and put these in a shallow serving bowl. If your chicory are particularly large, you may want to separate some of the leaves. Cut the apple into quarters, remove the core and slice the apple quarters fairly thinly. Peel and finely slice the onion. Roughly chop the mint and parsley leaves.

Toss the chicory, apple, onion, hazelnuts, cumin seeds and herbs together lightly. Scatter the beetroot on top of the salad and tumble gently through the salad. Spoon over a little of the dressing. Serve the rest of the dressing separately or cover and keep for other salads. It should last for a couple of days in the fridge.

**SERVES 4**

2 medium beetroot, each about 200g
20g blanched hazelnuts
½ tsp cumin seeds (optional)
2 chicory heads, trimmed
1 red eating apple
½ small red onion
small handful of fresh mint leaves
small handful of fresh flat-leaf parsley

**Dressing**
150g low-fat natural yoghurt
juice and finely grated zest of ½ lime
2 tsp runny honey

*122 calories per portion*

# WARM GRIDDLED VEGETABLES

*Salads don't have to be cold and in this simple dish charring the veg gives extra flavour without extra calories. For a main meal for two, serve with 125g sliced halloumi cheese – just pop it on to the griddle for a couple of minutes, turning halfway through the cooking time. Adding the halloumi to your meal will increase the calories per person by about 200 calories.*

**SERVES 2**

1 red pepper
1 yellow pepper
3 medium courgettes
1 medium red onion
2 tsp olive oil
freshly ground pepper

**Chilli dressing**
1 plump red chilli, finely diced
1 garlic clove, peeled and crushed
bunch of fresh coriander (about 10g), roughly chopped
1½ tsp extra virgin olive oil
1 tsp red wine vinegar

*148 calories per portion (without halloumi)*
*348 calories per portion (with halloumi)*

Place a large heavy-based griddle pan over a medium-high heat. Cut the peppers in half from top to bottom and remove the green stalk end and seeds. Cut peppers in half again to make 4 long quarters from each and put them in a large bowl.

Trim the courgettes and cut them into long, diagonal slices, about 1cm thick. Peel the red onion, leaving the root intact, and then cut into 8 wedges. Put the courgettes and onion in the bowl with the peppers and pour over the 2 teaspoons of olive oil. Season with lots of ground black pepper and toss the veg together well.

Scatter the vegetables on to the hot griddle and cook for 6–8 minutes, pressing with a spatula to flatten them on to the griddle. Turn once. The onions and courgettes will be ready before the peppers, so they can be transferred to a shallow serving dish as soon as they are tender and lightly charred. Continue cooking the peppers until they are softened. If your griddle isn't very big, cook the vegetables in batches so you don't overcrowd the pan.

While the vegetables are cooking, mix all the dressing ingredients until thoroughly combined. Add the cooked peppers to the serving dish with the onion and courgettes and toss lightly. Season with lots of ground black pepper, then spoon the dressing over the vegetables and tumble them gently until they are all coated. Serve warm.

*Top tip:* *If you don't fancy making the chilli dressing, this is also good served just with a dribble of good balsamic vinegar.*

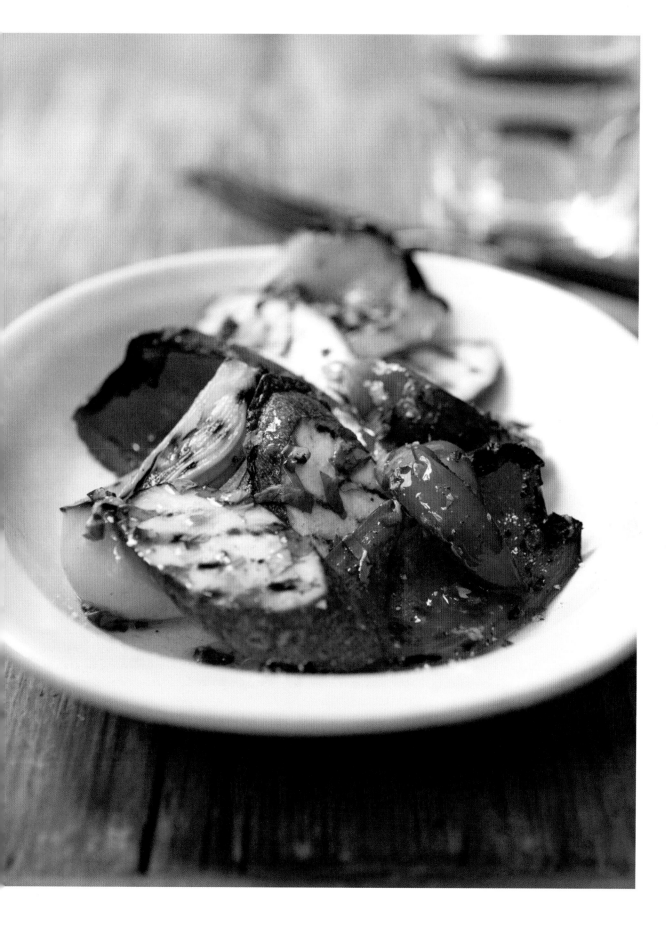

# FRUITY RICE SALAD

*This happy mix of sweet and savoury is spicy, satisfying and delivers every flavour combination you could want. You could even add a little chilli if you like a touch more heat. Lovely with grilled or barbecued meat or fish – or even some lamb chops when your diet is over.*

**SERVES 4 AS A LUNCH OR 6 AS AN ACCOMPANIMENT**

125g easy-cook wholegrain rice
2 tsp olive oil
½ medium red onion, finely chopped
1 tsp ground cumin
1 tsp ground coriander
½ tsp ground turmeric
2 tbsp cold water
freshly squeezed juice and finely grated zest of 1 small unwaxed lemon
1 small pineapple or half a medium pineapple, roughly 500g
½ cucumber
100g bunch of seedless red grapes
large handful of fresh coriander, roughly chopped

*202 calories per portion (if serving 4)*
*135 calories per portion (if serving 6)*

Half fill a medium saucepan with water and bring it to the boil. Add the rice, stir well and bring it back to the boil, then cook for 10 minutes or until tender. If you prefer to use a wholegrain rice that isn't the easy-cook kind, follow the packet instructions.

While the rice is cooking, prepare the other ingredients. Heat the oil in a small non-stick frying pan and fry the onion for 3–4 minutes until it's starting to soften, stirring occasionally. Add the cumin, coriander and turmeric and cook together for 30 seconds, stirring constantly. Add the water and cook for 2 minutes more or until the water has evaporated, stirring constantly. Take the pan off the heat and add the lemon juice and zest, then stir well.

Put the pineapple on a board and cut off the leaves and skin. Cut it in half and then quarters lengthways and remove the tough central core. Cut the pineapple flesh into rough 2cm chunks – you should end up with about 200g of prepared pineapple. Cut the cucumber into 1.5cm cubes and halve the grapes. Put the pineapple and grapes in a large serving bowl.

Drain the cooked rice and rinse in a sieve under running water until cold. Drain again, tip it into the pan with onion and spices and stir well until the rice is coated in the spices. Stir into the bowl with the fruit, add the chopped coriander and mix thoroughly.

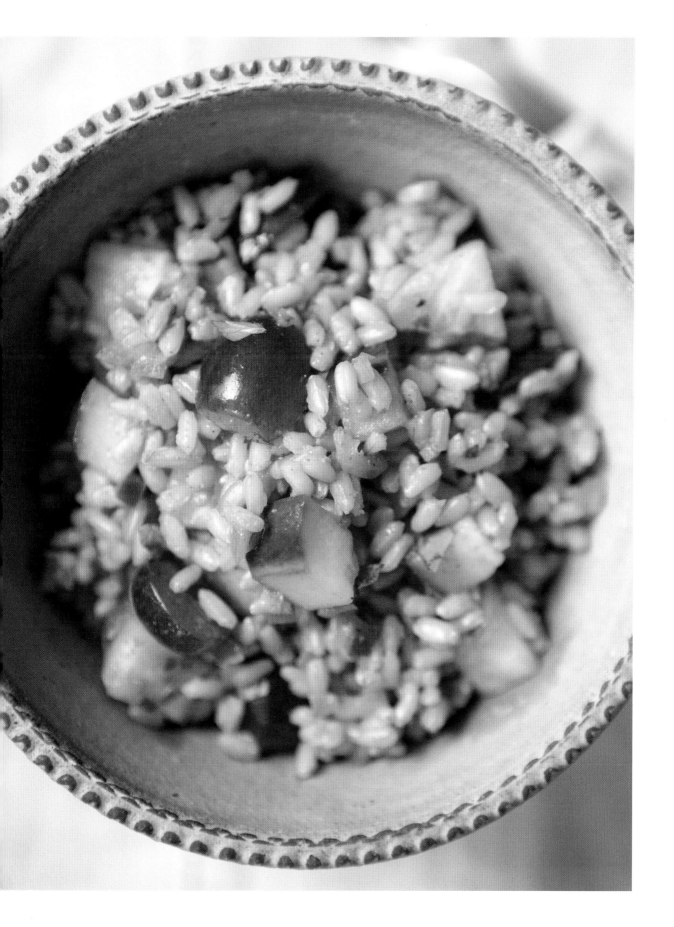

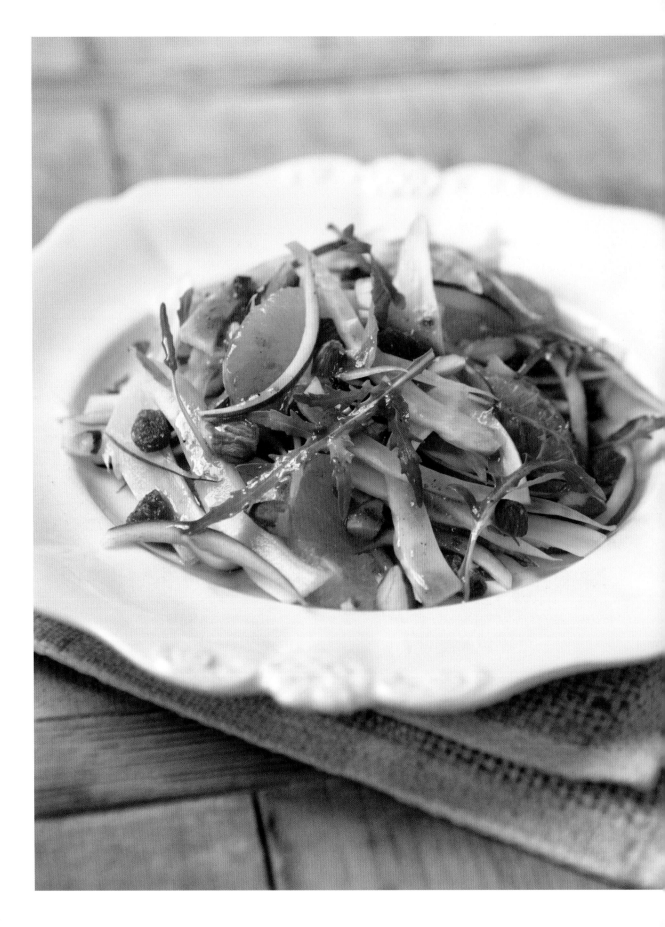

# FENNEL AND ORANGE SALAD
# WITH HARISSA DRESSING

*We've come to love our salads and this is a particularly tasty one – just right with a piece of grilled fish. The danger with salads can be that you drench your lovely healthy veg in oil, which is high in calories, so we're getting very clever with dressings. We've found ways of adding lots of flavour without too much oil, and this harissa dressing is one of our favourites.*

Trim the fennel and cut off any damaged parts. Place the fennel on its side and cut it into very thin slices from top to bottom. Put the fennel in a large serving bowl.

Cut a thin slice off the top of each orange so they sit flat. Stand each orange on a board and cut away the peel and pith with a sharp knife. Carefully cut between the segments and flip out the orange pieces into the same bowl as the fennel. Add the onion, then sprinkle the rocket, almonds and sultanas on top and toss everything together.

To make the dressing, put the harissa paste, garlic, coriander, vinegar, honey and a couple of twists of freshly ground black pepper in a small bowl and stir until thoroughly combined.

Slowly add the oil, just a few drops at a time, stirring vigorously with a spoon or a fork between each addition. The dressing will thicken a little as you mix it. Pour the dressing over the salad, toss lightly together and serve immediately.

**SERVES 2 AS A MAIN COURSE AND 4 AS AN ACCOMPANIMENT**

1 medium fennel bulb
2 large oranges
½ small red onion, cut into thin wedges
50g bag of rocket leaves
25g roasted salted almonds, roughly chopped
25g sultanas

**Harissa dressing**
1 tsp harissa paste (preferably rose harissa)
1 small garlic clove, peeled and crushed
good pinch of ground coriander
1½ tsp white wine vinegar
1 tsp runny honey
1 tbsp olive oil
freshly ground black pepper

---

*253 calories per portion (if serving 2)*
*124 calories per portion (if serving 4)*

# SI AND DAVE'S WEIGHT-LOSS TIPS

––––––––

We all love a takeaway once in a while, but they can be real diet busters as they are often laden with fat, not to mention the rice, bread and so on.

––––––––

Try our very own 'fakeaways' instead and you could save money and calories. We've reduced the fat but included plenty of spice and flavour so they taste like the food from your local restaurant but with fewer calories.

––––––––

Cook your fakeaways with as little fat as possible and trim any fat off the meat. Thicken the sauce with cornflour to give that rich texture.

––––––––

If you do want to order in, choose tandoori or other grilled dishes as they will be less fattening. Ask the restaurant not to dress the tandoori with ghee, though. Looks nice but adds loads of calories.

––––––––

Don't overdo the rice. A serving of about 50g (uncooked) per person is plenty when you're watching the calories.

––––––––

# FAKEAWAYS

"I've learned you can deliver great taste without diet damage."

*Dave*

# SWEET AND SOUR CHICKEN

*This is exactly like your favourite sweet and sour from the local down the road, but with fewer calories. Proves that a diet doesn't have to be all about denial.*

**SERVES 4**

2 boneless, skinless chicken breasts
2 tbsp sunflower oil
1 medium onion, cut
into 12 wedges
2 peppers, red, green, orange or
yellow, deseeded and cut into
chunks of about 3cm
225g can of water chestnuts
2 garlic cloves, peeled and crushed
25g chunk of fresh root ginger,
peeled and finely grated
freshly ground black pepper

**Sauce**

425g can of pineapple chunks
in natural juice
2 tbsp cornflour
150ml water
2 tbsp dark soy sauce
2 tbsp white wine vinegar
2 tbsp soft light brown sugar
2 tbsp tomato ketchup
½ tsp dried chilli flakes

*288 calories per portion (without rice)*

To make the sauce, drain the pineapple in a sieve over a bowl and keep all the juice – you should have about 150ml. Put the cornflour in a large bowl and stir in 3 tablespoons of the pineapple juice to make a smooth paste. Add the remaining juice and the water, then stir in the soy sauce, vinegar, sugar, ketchup and chilli flakes until thoroughly combined. Set aside.

Cut each chicken breast into 8 or 9 even pieces. Heat a tablespoon of the oil in a large non-stick frying pan or wok and stir-fry the onion and peppers for 2 minutes over a high heat. Drain the water chestnuts and cut them in half horizontally.

Add the remaining oil and the chicken to the pan and stir-fry for 2 minutes until coloured on all sides. Add the garlic, ginger, pineapple chunks and water chestnuts and stir-fry for 30–60 seconds.

Give the cornflour and pineapple mixture a good stir and add it to the pan with the chicken and vegetables. Stir well, season with some ground black pepper and bring to a simmer. Cook for 4–6 minutes until the sauce is thickened and glossy and the chicken is tender and cooked throughout, turning the chicken and vegetables a few times. Serve with a small portion of rice.

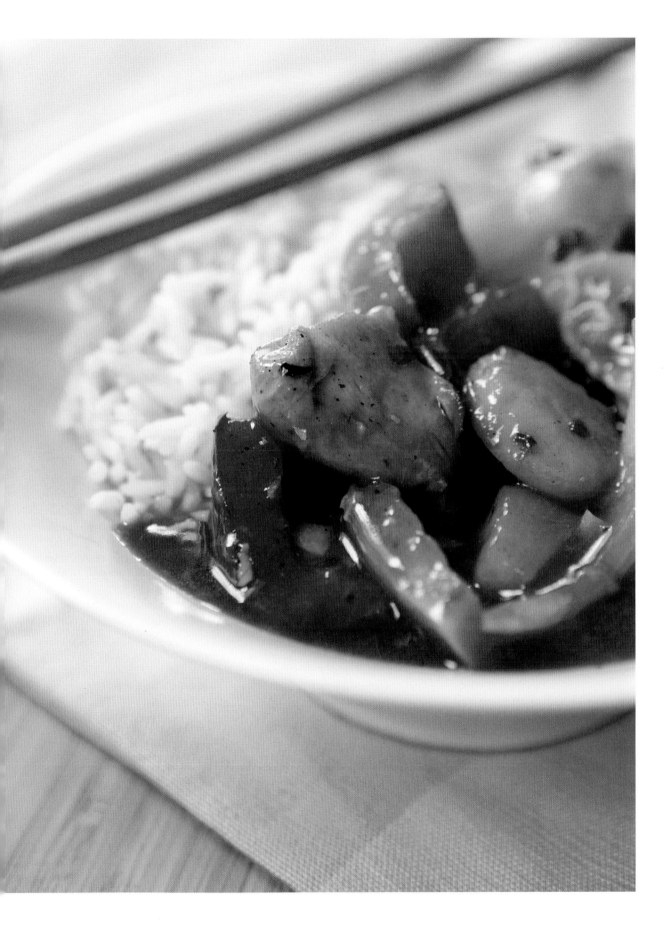

# CHICKEN KORMA

*Rich, creamy chicken korma is usually forbidden territory if you're watching your weight, but we'd hate you to miss out so we've come up with our korma-lite. A good all-round curry recipe, this is much lower in fat than the usual restaurant version but still fab to eat. Add extra chilli if you like.*

### SERVES 4

4 fairly small boneless, skinless chicken breasts (about 600g)
25g low-fat natural yoghurt
1 tbsp sunflower oil
2 large onions, chopped (400g prepared weight)
4 garlic cloves, peeled and sliced
20g chunk of fresh root ginger, peeled and finely grated
12 cardamom pods, seeds crushed
1 tbsp ground cumin
1 tbsp ground coriander
½ heaped tsp ground turmeric
¼ tsp hot chilli powder
1 bay leaf
4 whole cloves
1 tbsp plain flour
small pinch of saffron
2 tsp caster sugar
½ tsp fine sea salt, plus extra to season
300ml cold water
3 tbsp double cream
freshly ground black pepper
fresh coriander, roughly torn, to garnish (optional)

*294 calories per portion (without rice)*

Cut each chicken breast into 8 or 9 bite-sized pieces, season with black pepper and put them in a non-metallic bowl. Stir in the yoghurt, cover with cling film and chill for a minimum of 30 minutes but ideally 2–6 hours.

Heat the oil in a large, non-stick saucepan and add the onions, garlic and ginger. Cover and cook over a low heat for 15 minutes until very soft and lightly coloured. Stir the onions occasionally so they don't start to stick.

Once the onions are softened, stir in the crushed cardamom seeds, cumin, coriander, turmeric, chilli powder and bay leaf. Pinch off the ends of the cloves into the pan and throw away the stalks. Cook the spices with the onions for 5 minutes, stirring constantly.

Stir in the flour, saffron, sugar and ½ a teaspoon of salt, then slowly pour the water into the pan, stirring constantly. Bring to a gentle simmer, then cover and cook for 10 minutes, stirring occasionally. Remove the pan from the heat, take out the bay leaf and blitz the onion mixture with a stick blender until it is as smooth as possible. You can do this in a food processor if you prefer, but let the mixture cool slightly first. The sauce can now be used right away or cooled, covered and chilled until 10 minutes before serving.

Drain the chicken in a colander over the sink, shaking it a few times – you want the meat to have just a light coating of yoghurt. Place a non-stick frying pan on the heat, add the sauce and bring it to a simmer. Add the chicken pieces and cream and cook for about 10 minutes or until the chicken is tender and cooked through, stirring regularly. Exactly how long the chicken takes will depend on the size of your pieces, so check a piece after 8 minutes – there should be no pink remaining.

Adjust the seasoning to taste, spoon into a warmed serving dish and serve garnished with fresh coriander if you like.

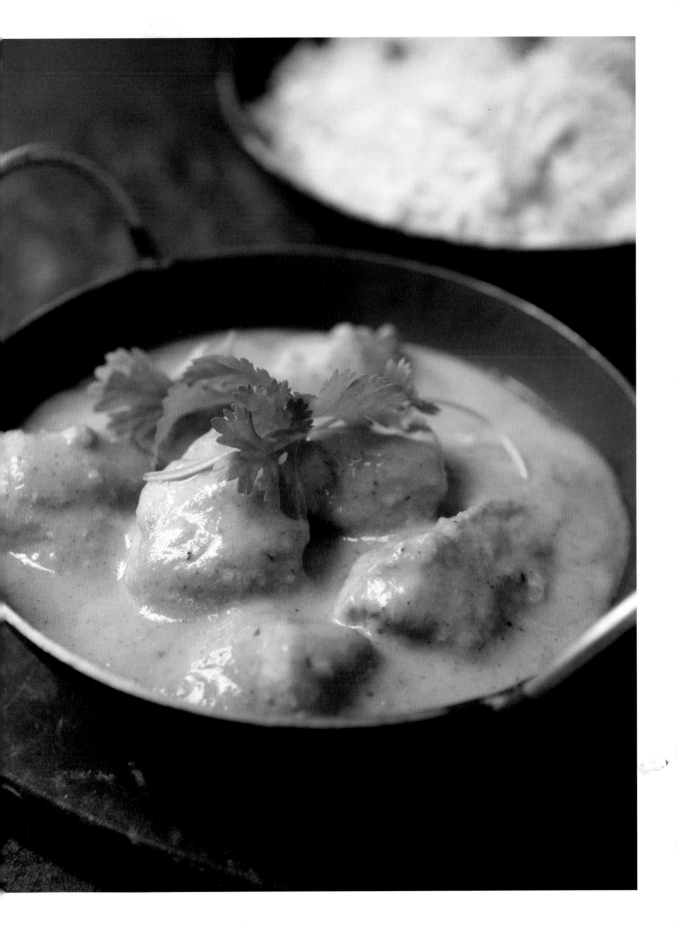

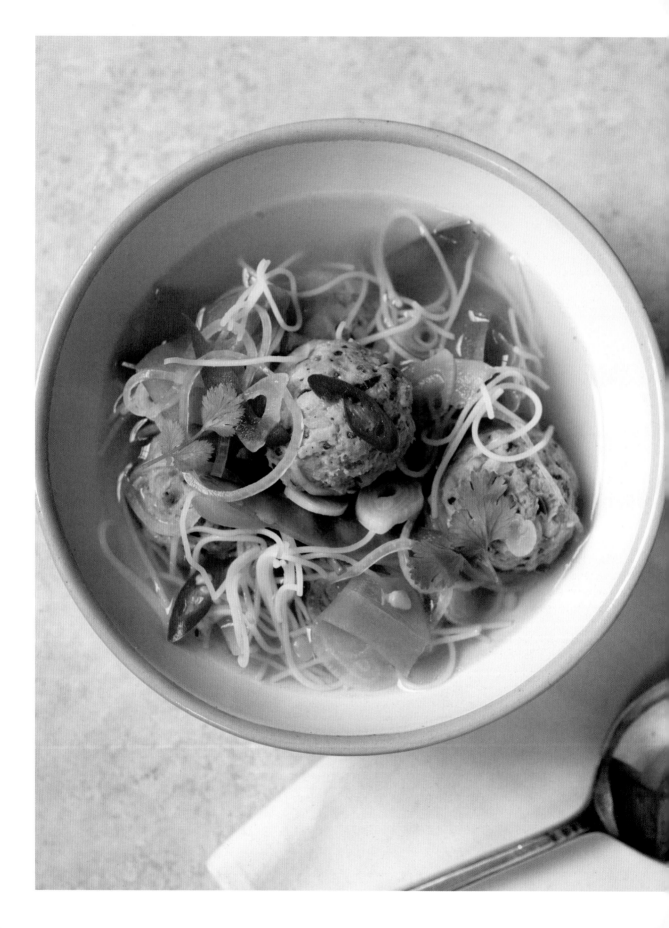

# FRAGRANT PORK AND PRAWN NOODLE BROTH

*Hot and spicy, this delicious broth contains lots of vegetables as well as pork and prawn meatballs and is light but filling. Follow the recipe to the letter and you'll find it works brilliantly. We know there's a long list of ingredients, but you should be able to find them all in your local supermarket. Cut down on chilli if you like a more delicate flavour.*

To make the broth base, pour the water into a large saucepan and add the stock cube. Bring to a simmer, stirring to dissolve the cube. Roughly chop the lemongrass stalks and add them to the pan. Split 2 of the chillies lengthways almost all the way through and pop them in the pan too.

Add the lime leaves, half the sliced shallots and all the ginger and garlic. Bring the broth to a low simmer and cook gently for 20 minutes. Remove the pan from the heat and leave to stand for about 30 minutes while you make the pork and prawn balls.

Put the pork mince, prawns, chopped shallot, garlic, chilli (deseed it first if you like), cornflour, salt and lots of freshly ground black pepper in a food processor and blend to make a thick, slightly textured purée. Add the coriander leaves and give it another quick blitz until just combined. Take out the processor blade, then roll the pork and prawn mixture into 20 small balls and put them on a large dinner plate.

Strain the infused stock through a sieve into a clean pan. Stir in the remaining sliced shallot, lime juice and nam pla. Slice the remaining 2 bird's eye chillies very finely and add them to the pan. Bring to a gentle simmer and add the pork balls.

Return to a simmer and cook for 5 minutes, allowing the liquid to bubble gently. While the pork balls are simmering, cut the carrots into long ribbons using a vegetable peeler. Deseed the peppers and slice them thinly, and wipe and slice the mushrooms. Trim the mangetout and cut them in half diagonally. Stir the carrot strips, mushrooms, mangetout, peppers and noodles into the broth and simmer for 3–4 minutes or until the pork balls are cooked through and the vegetables and noodles are just tender, stirring occasionally.

Ladle the broth into deep bowls, making sure everyone has their fair share of pork and prawn balls. Scatter the coriander on top and serve.

## SERVES 4

2 litres cold water
1 chicken stock cube
2 lemongrass stalks
4 red bird's eye chillies
6 kaffir lime leaves, dried or fresh
2 long shallots, thinly sliced
50g fresh root ginger, peeled and thinly sliced
4 garlic cloves, peeled and halved lengthways
4 tbsp fresh lime juice (1½ limes)
3 tbsp nam pla (Thai fish sauce)
2 medium carrots, peeled
1 small red pepper
1 small yellow pepper
150g chestnut mushrooms
150g mangetout
50g fine vermicelli rice noodles
large handful of fresh coriander, roughly torn, to garnish

**Pork and prawn balls**
250g lean minced pork
100g cooked peeled prawns, thawed if frozen
½ long shallot (about 25g), peeled and finely chopped
2 garlic cloves, finely chopped
1 bird's eye chilli, finely chopped
1 tbsp cornflour
¼ tsp fine sea salt
2 tbsp finely chopped fresh coriander leaves
freshly ground black pepper

*270 calories per portion*

# LAMB, SPINACH AND POTATO CURRY

*This is a low-cal version of Dave's favourite curry – saag gosht – because he couldn't bear to give it up. If you are running short of time, cut out the fresh garlic, ginger and chilli – the curry will still taste great. The recipe contains potatoes so there is no need to serve it with extra rice.*

**SERVES 6**

600g lamb leg steaks
(about 4 steaks)
1 tbsp sunflower oil
2 large onions, roughly chopped
4 large garlic cloves,
peeled and roughly chopped
25g chunk of fresh root ginger,
peeled and roughly chopped
1 plump fresh red chilli, roughly
chopped (deseeded if you like)
75g medium or mild curry paste
(depending on your taste)
400g can of chopped tomatoes
350g potatoes, preferably Maris
Pipers, peeled and cut into
3cm chunks
450ml water
2 bay leaves
1 tsp flaked sea salt, plus extra for
seasoning the meat
1 tsp caster sugar
3 ripe medium tomatoes, quartered
100g young spinach leaves
freshly ground black pepper

*293 calories per portion*

Trim the lamb of any hard fat and cut the meat into rough chunks of about 3cm. Season with salt and pepper. Heat a teaspoon of the oil in a large non-stick frying pan and fry the lamb in 2 batches until lightly coloured on all sides. Transfer the lamb to a plate as soon as each batch is browned.

Heat the remaining oil in a large flameproof casserole dish and add the onions. Cook over a medium heat for 6–8 minutes until they're softened and lightly browned, stirring regularly. Turn down the heat, add the garlic, ginger, chilli and curry paste and cook for 5 minutes more, stirring frequently.

Remove from the heat and blitz the onion mixture with a stick blender until blended to a purée. Or you can let the mixture cool for a few minutes, then blend it in a food processor before tipping it back into the casserole. Return the casserole to the hob over a medium heat. Preheat the oven to 190°C/Fan 170°C/Gas 5.

Add the browned lamb to the spiced onion purée in the dish and cook over a gentle heat for 2–3 minutes, stirring. Add the canned chopped tomatoes, potatoes, water, bay leaves, teaspoon of salt and the sugar. Bring everything to a gentle simmer, then cover with a lid and place the casserole in the oven for 1 hour and 30 minutes or until the lamb is tender and the sauce has thickened. Check after 1 hour and give the contents of the casserole dish a good stir.

Take the dish out of the oven and remove the lid. Stir in the quartered tomatoes and spinach leaves. Cover once more and return to the oven for a further 5 minutes or until the tomatoes are soft and the spinach has wilted. Serve hot with some spoonfuls of fat-free yoghurt if you fancy.

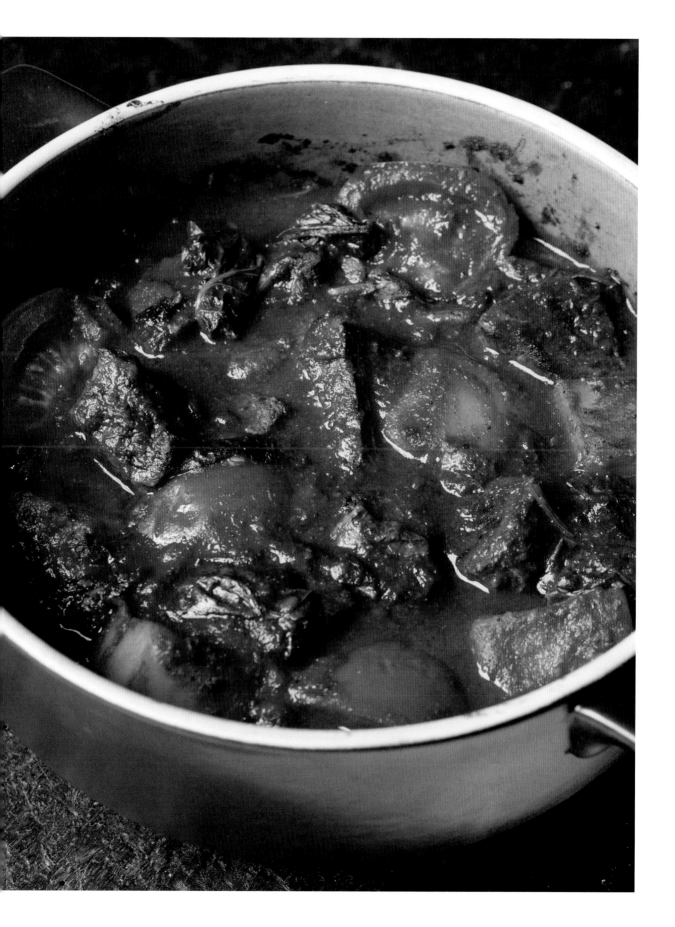

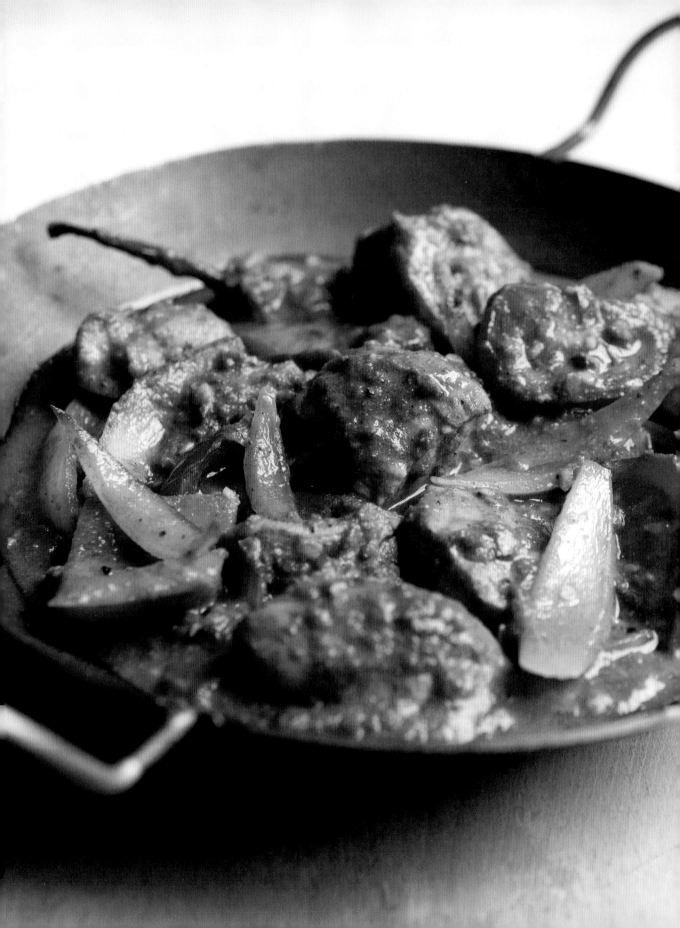

# CHICKEN JALFREZI

*A culinary triumph for curry-loving dieters – what's not to like? We've reworked this classic to encourage your ever-decreasing waistline, so get shopping and chopping.*

Finely chop 4 of the chillies – deseed a couple or all of them first if you don't like very spicy food. Split the other 2 chillies from stalk to tip on 1 side without opening or removing the seeds. Cut each chicken breast into 7 or 8 bite-sized chunks.

Heat a tablespoon of the oil in a large, fairly deep, non-stick frying pan (or wok) over a high heat. Add the garlic, chopped chillies, chopped tomatoes, cumin, garam masala, turmeric, sugar and salt, then stir-fry for 3–4 minutes until the vegetables soften. Don't let the garlic or spices burn or they will add a bitter flavour to the sauce.

Next, add the chicken pieces and whole chillies and cook for 3 minutes, turning the chicken regularly. Pour over the 200ml of water, stir in the yoghurt and reduce the heat only slightly – you want the sauce to simmer. Cook for about 8 minutes, stirring occasionally until the chicken is tender and cooked through and the sauce has reduced by about a third. The yoghurt may separate to begin with but will disappear into the sauce.

While the chicken is cooking, heat the remaining tablespoon of oil in a clean pan and stir-fry the onion and pepper over a high heat for 3–4 minutes until lightly browned. Add the quartered tomatoes and fry for 2–3 minutes more, stirring until the vegetables are just tender. Mix the cornflour with the tablespoon of water to form a smooth paste.

When the chicken is cooked, stir in the cornflour mixture and simmer for a few seconds until the sauce thickens, stirring constantly. Remove from the heat, add the hot stir-fried vegetables and toss together lightly. Serve immediately. And just in case you were wondering – don't eat the whole chillies!

## SERVES 4

6 long green chillies
4 boneless, skinless chicken breasts
2 tbsp sunflower oil
2 garlic cloves, peeled and finely chopped
3 ripe tomatoes, chopped
1 tbsp ground cumin
1 tbsp garam masala
1 tsp ground turmeric
1 tbsp caster sugar
1 tsp flaked sea salt
200ml cold water
2 tbsp low-fat natural yoghurt
1 medium onion, cut into 12 wedges
1 green pepper, deseeded and cut into rough 3cm chunks
2 tomatoes, quartered
2 tsp cornflour
1 tbsp water

*279 calories per portion*

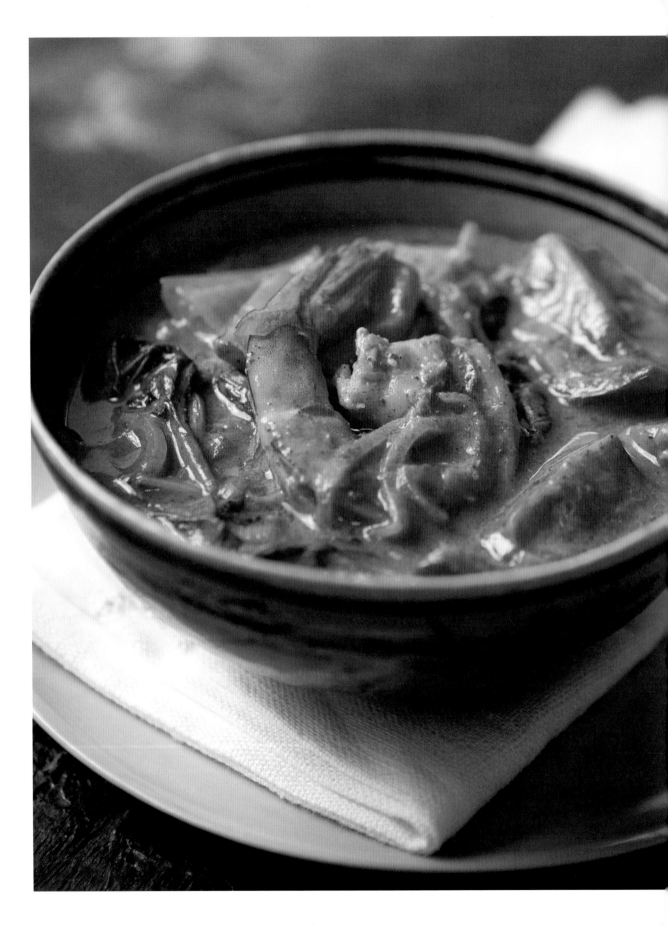

# COCONUT PRAWN CURRY

*This is an adaptation of one of our Keralan favourites. A lot of curries tend to be very rich because they are thickened with coconut milk or cream, but there are alternatives and we've found good reduced-fat coconut milk. A little goes a long way too, so you can get away with using less than usual but still get the flavour.*

Put the curry paste, 1 tablespoon of water, onion and pepper in a large non-stick frying pan. Cook over a low heat for 4–5 minutes, stirring regularly until the onion is softened.

Add the mango chutney, tomatoes and coconut milk and bring to a simmer. Cook for 4 minutes, stirring occasionally until the tomatoes are soft but still holding their shape. Mix the cornflour and 1 tablespoon of water to make a smooth paste. Add this to the coconut sauce and cook for 30 seconds or so, stirring constantly until the sauce thickens.

Stir in the prawns and spinach leaves and cook for 2–3 minutes or until the prawns are hot and the spinach is softened, stirring regularly. If you're using raw prawns, make sure they are completely pink before serving.

Serve the curry with a small portion of freshly cooked basmati rice.

**SERVES 2**

2 tbsp medium curry paste
2 tbsp cold water
1 medium onion, halved and
finely sliced
1 orange or yellow pepper, deseeded
and cut into rough 3cm chunks
1 tbsp mango chutney
3 large ripe tomatoes, quartered
200ml half-fat coconut milk
2 tsp cornflour
200g cooked or raw peeled king
prawns, thawed if frozen
100g baby spinach leaves

*254 calories per portion (without rice)*

# VERY EASY THAI CHICKEN AND COCONUT CURRY

*We like our curry spicy and hot, so cut the curry paste to level tablespoons if you prefer your food a little milder. Don't be tempted to leave out the nam pla. It might sound funny but it adds that authentic Thai flavour to the curry and you can find it in most large supermarkets and delis now.*

**SERVES 4**

1 tbsp sunflower oil
3 boneless, skinless chicken breasts, cut into thin slices
1 large red pepper, deseeded and cut into thin strips
1 large yellow pepper, deseeded and cut into thin strips
400ml can of half-fat coconut milk
250ml cold water, plus 2 tbsp
2 heaped tbsp Thai green or red curry paste
6 dried or fresh kaffir lime leaves
4 tsp nam pla (Thai fish sauce)
1 tsp caster sugar
150g mangetout peas, trimmed
2 tbsp cornflour
small handful of fresh coriander, roughly torn (optional)
small handful of fresh basil leaves, roughly torn (optional)

Heat the oil in a large non-stick saucepan, frying pan or wok. Stir-fry the chicken and peppers for 1 minute. Pour over the coconut milk and add the 250ml of water, curry paste, lime leaves, fish sauce and caster sugar. Bring to a gentle simmer and cook for 5 minutes, stirring regularly.

Add the mangetout and return to a simmer. Mix the cornflour with the remaining 2 tablespoons of cold water and stir into the pan. Cook for another 2–3 minutes until the vegetables are tender and the spiced coconut milk has thickened, stirring frequently. Serve the curry in deep bowls, scattered with fresh coriander or basil if using. By the way – don't eat the lime leaves.

*286 calories per portion (without rice)*

**Top tip:** *Serve this curry with jasmine rice or basmati rice. Aim to cook no more than 50g per person, so 200g in all. Press the freshly boiled rice into a 200ml metal pudding basin or dariole mould that you've oiled lightly and lined with cling film, then turn out into the bowls before adding the hot curry. You only need 1 basin or mould as you can reuse it for all the servings*

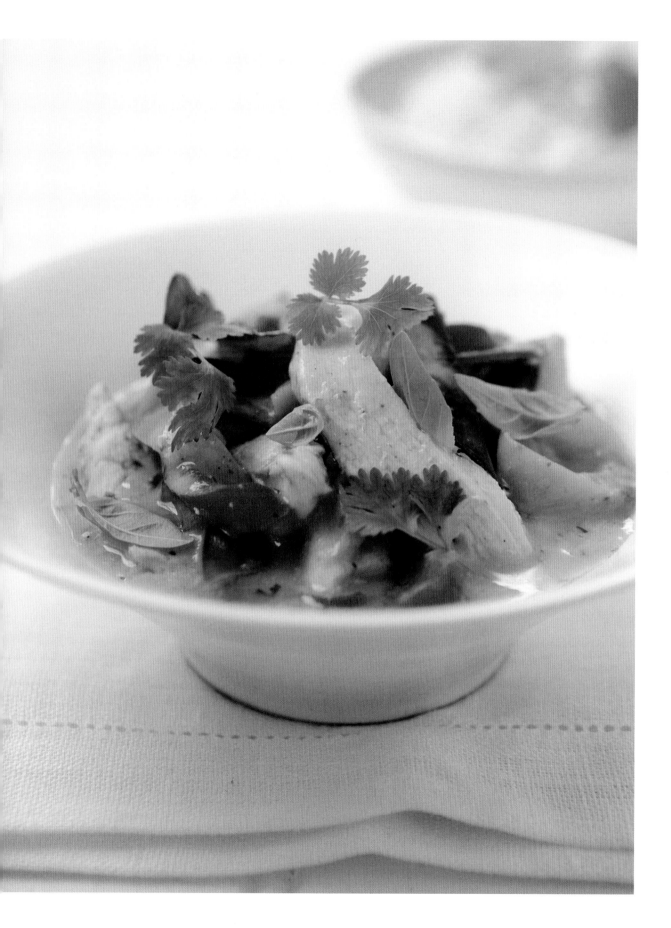

# SI AND DAVE'S WEIGHT-LOSS TIPS

———————

We've said it before and we'll say it again, cook just a 50g portion of rice to have with your meal. It won't look much if you're used to huge portions, but if you fill the rest of your plate with lots of colourful vegetables or salad, you will hardly notice.

———————

The idea of many pasta dishes is that the pasta adds bulk so you don't need so much of the sauce. When you're dieting, reverse this so you have less of the pasta and more of the good stuff.

———————

In dishes such as risotto it's not the rice that's the problem but the fat you add to it. Have a go at making our risotto which is lower in fat than usual – you're going to love it.

———————

Buy tomato-based sauces if you like, but check the calorie count on the label. Some of them are higher in calories than others.

———————

Bulk out home-made sauces with extra vegetables, such as peppers and aubergine. Whiz them up if you like a smooth sauce.

———————

Serve some extra protein like chicken or prawns with your pasta dish so you need less of the carbs.

———————

# PASTA & RICE

"We used to just chuck handfuls of pasta or rice into the pan. Now we weigh it so we don't eat too much."

*Si*

# HOME-MADE
# BUTTERNUT SQUASH TORTELLINI

*Didn't think you could eat stuffed pasta did you? Well, this recipe uses a gyoza dumpling dough, rather than a traditional home-made egg pasta, and could save you a whopping 240 calories or so for the recipe as a whole, and up to 60 calories a portion. The dough is much easier and quicker to roll than traditional pasta and makes beautiful tortellini. You can use the same recipe to make ravioli, lasagne or tagliatelle too.*

**SERVES 4**

300g strong white flour, plus extra
for rolling
½ tsp fine salt
200ml boiling water

**Filling**

500g butternut squash
(½ small squash)
1 tsp olive oil
1 small red onion
3 tbsp quick-cook polenta
25g Pecorino or Parmesan
cheese, finely grated
¼ tsp freshly grated nutmeg
flaked sea salt
freshly ground black pepper

**Sauce**

3 tbsp half-fat crème fraiche
handful fresh basil leaves,
roughly torn
2 big handfuls of baby
spinach leaves

*389 calories per portion*

First make the dough. Sift the flour and mix in the salt, then stir in the boiling water with chopsticks or a knife until a ball forms. If the dough seems too wet, add a bit more flour; if it's too dry, add more boiling water. Cover the dough and leave it to stand and cool for about an hour. Meanwhile, you can get on with the filling.

Preheat the oven to 200°C/Fan 180°C/Gas 6. Peel the butternut squash and cut it into rough 4cm chunks. Put these in a large bowl and toss with ½ tsp of the oil, a couple of pinches of salt and lots of freshly ground black pepper. Scatter over a large baking tray and roast for 25 minutes until just tender when pierced with a skewer.

While the squash is cooking, halve and finely slice the onion. Put the slices in the bowl used for the squash, add the remaining oil and toss well. Scatter over the top of the squash after the 25 minutes cooking time and roast together for 10 minutes more.

Tip the hot vegetables back into the mixing bowl and leave to cool for 5 minutes. Add the polenta and blitz with a stick blender (or in a food processor if you prefer) to make a thick, orange purée. Set aside to cool for about an hour, then stir in the grated cheese and nutmeg. Adjust salt and pepper to taste.

Place the dough on a lightly floured surface and knead for 5 minutes until it's very elastic. You can do this in a food mixer with a dough hook if you like. Take a third of the dough and roll it out very thinly on a floured surface, stretching and turning it as you go. Cut out 10 circles with a 9cm round pastry cutter, stacking the discs with a dusting of flour between them to stop them sticking. Continue until all the dough is used up – you can't re-roll this dough.

Take a disc of dough and lay it flat in the palm of your hand. Place a heaped teaspoon of filling in the middle, dip your finger in water and brush it around the edge. Fold the pastry over and, gently squeezing out the excess air, press the edges firmly to form a semi-circular shape. Bring the two ends of the crescent round in front of the filling and dampen one end with a little cold water. Press firmly together to seal and create the tortellini shape. Set aside on a floured plate while you make the rest.

Half fill a very large saucepan with cold water and bring to the boil. Drop the tortellini gently into the hot water and bring it back to the boil. Cook for 5 minutes or until the pasta is tender, stirring occasionally. Drain the pasta in a colander, leaving just 3–4 tablespoons of the cooking liquid in the pan to form the base for the sauce.

Tip the pasta back into the saucepan and add the crème fraiche, basil and spinach leaves. Season well with the chilli flakes and some freshly ground black pepper, then toss together over a low heat until the spinach wilts. Divide the tortellini between warmed plates to serve.

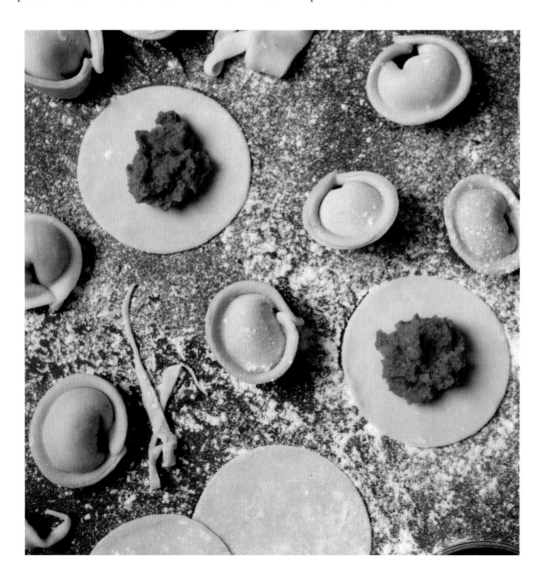

# BEACHSIDE PAELLA

*We cooked this on a beach in Northumberland and some said it was the best paella they'd ever tasted – dieting or not. You know what? We have to agree.*

**SERVES 6**

1 tbsp olive oil
6 boneless, skinless chicken thighs, cut in half
75g chorizo (we like picante) skinned and cut into 5mm slices
2 medium onions, peeled and chopped
1 red pepper, quartered, deseeded and sliced
1 yellow pepper, quartered, deseeded and sliced
150g green beans, trimmed and cut into 2cm lengths
3 garlic cloves, peeled and crushed
2 tsp smoked paprika
2 good pinches of saffron threads
1 bay leaf
175g paella rice (medium-grain rice)
1 litre hot chicken stock, made with 1 chicken stock cube
500g live mussels, well scrubbed and beards removed
1 medium squid, cleaned and sliced into rings or 225g prepared squid rings
12 raw king prawns, peeled or shells on, thawed if frozen
flaked sea salt
freshly ground black pepper
lemon wedges, for squeezing

*358 calories per portion*

Heat the oil in a 38cm paella pan – ideally non-stick. A paella pan is best, but if you don't have one, use a very wide, shallow non-stick saucepan, flameproof casserole dish or sauté pan.

Place the pan over a medium heat. Season the chicken thighs with salt and black pepper and fry them for about 5 minutes, turning every now and then until lightly coloured. Add the chorizo and cook for 30 seconds more, turning once. Transfer the chicken and chorizo to a large heatproof bowl with a slotted spoon, leaving the fat in the pan.

Add the onions to the pan and fry gently for 4–5 minutes until softened and very lightly browned, stirring occasionally. Add the peppers and green beans to the onions and cook for 2 minutes until they are beginning to soften. Stir in the garlic, smoked paprika, saffron, bay leaf and rice and cook for 1–2 minutes until the rice is glistening all over.

Return the chicken and chorizo to the pan, along with any juices. Stir well, then pour in the chicken stock and season with black pepper. Stir once or twice and bring to a simmer over a medium heat. Cook for 12 minutes, stirring occasionally.

Tip the mussels into the partly cooked rice mixture and stir once more, making sure they are well tucked into the hot rice and steaming liquid. Return to a simmer and cook for 3 minutes or until most of the mussels have opened, stirring occasionally.

Scatter the squid and prawns over the top of the paella and stir well. Continue cooking for 4–5 minutes until the squid and prawns are cooked, the rice is tender and almost all the liquid has been absorbed. The prawns should be completely pink when cooked.

It's important not to keep stirring after the squid and prawns are added – you want the rice to become lightly browned and a bit sticky at the sides of the pan as this adds flavour. Keep an eye on the heat though, as you don't want the rice to burn. Add a splash more water if the paella begins to look very dry before the rice is ready. Pick out any mussels that haven't opened by the end of the cooking time and chuck them away. Serve hot with lemon wedges for squeezing.

Top tip:

*Make sure you wash and scrub your mussels really well, knocking off any barnacles which might be hitch-hiking a ride. Throw away any mussels that have broken or damaged shells. Tap any that are open on the edge of the sink. They should close, but if they don't, throw them away as they are probably dead.*

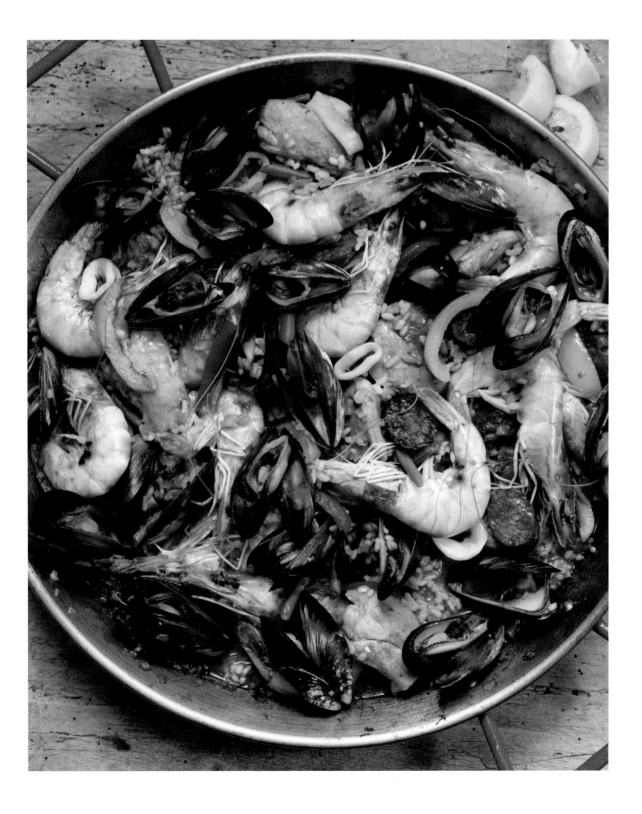

# CHILLI LEMON TUNA AND BROCCOLI SPAGHETTI

*A quick and easy lunch or supper dish that really hits the spot. Make sure you use very fresh tuna steaks, especially if you like them a little rare, or you can swap the tuna for salmon steaks or even white fish fillets if you prefer. Note the amount of pasta and don't overdo it.*

**SERVES 2**

150g tenderstem broccoli
100g dried spaghetti
1 tsp dried chilli flakes
½ tsp flaked sea salt
½ tsp coarsely ground black pepper
2 very fresh tuna steaks
(about 150g each)
1 tbsp olive oil
100g cherry tomatoes, halved
freshly squeezed juice of 1 lemon
1 tsp chilli oil
3 heaped tbsp flat-leaf parsley,
roughly chopped
lemon wedges, for squeezing
(optional)

*472 calories per portion*

Half fill a large saucepan with water and bring it to the boil. Trim the broccoli and cut each stem into 3 pieces, leaving the heads intact. Add the spaghetti to the boiling water, return to the boil and cook for 10 minutes, stirring occasionally. Add the broccoli to the same pan and cook for 2 minutes more.

While the pasta is cooking, mix the dried chilli flakes, salt and pepper together in a small bowl. Sprinkle the mixture lightly over both sides of the tuna and set aside. Pour the oil into a large non-stick frying pan and place over a medium-high heat. You need a large frying pan because you will be tossing the drained pasta in the same pan. Fry the tuna steaks for 2–3 minutes on each side, depending on how thick they are. If you like your tuna rare, cook for 1½ minutes on each side.

Drain the pasta and broccoli in a colander. Put the tuna on warmed plates and add the drained spaghetti, broccoli, tomatoes, lemon juice, chilli oil and parsley to the frying pan.

Cook for 2 minutes, tossing with 2 wooden spoons until the pasta is lightly coated with the spices from the pan and the tomatoes are softened but still holding their shape. Divide the spaghetti between the plates using tongs or a couple of forks. Add some extra lemon wedges for squeezing if you like. Serve right away while it's all lovely and hot.

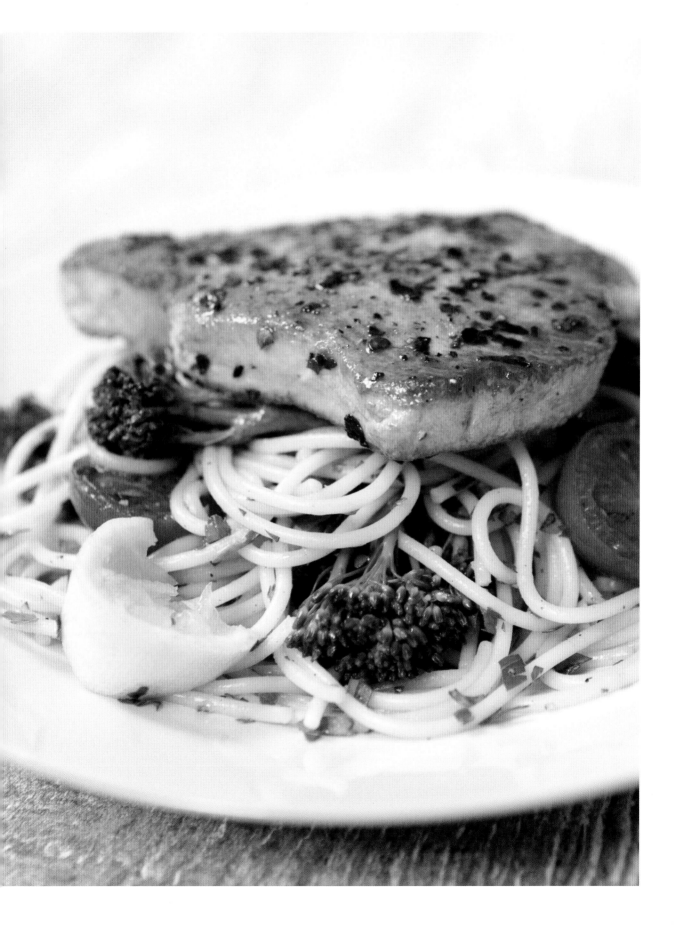

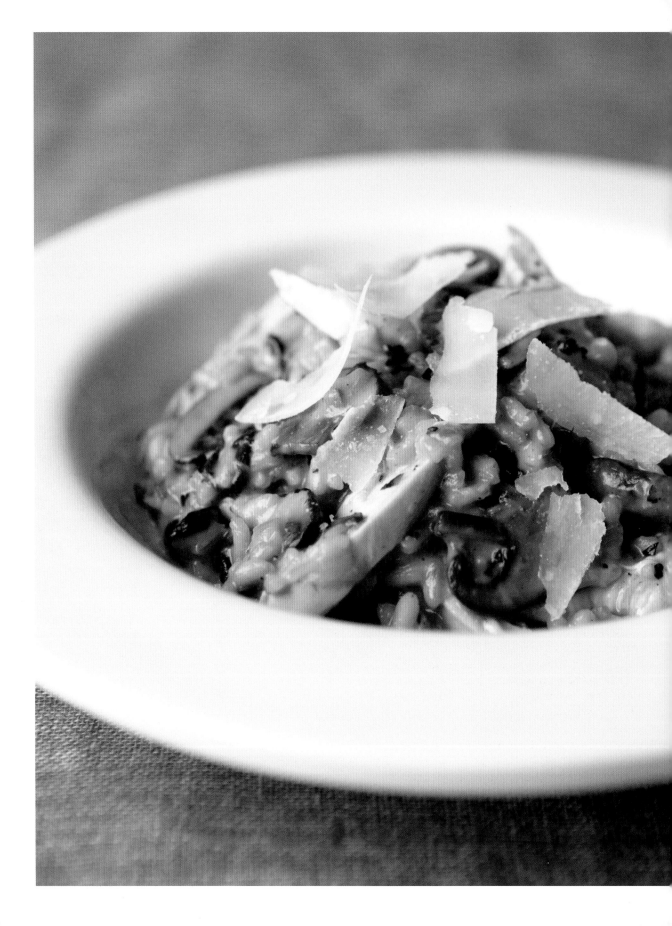

# CHICKEN AND MUSHROOM RISOTTO

*Bet you didn't think you could eat risotto and still shed the pounds? Well, you didn't reckon with our clever cooking skills. We've radically reduced the fat content of a normal risotto while sacrificing little of the flavour and texture. A classic mid-week supper.*

Put the dried mushrooms in a small heatproof bowl and pour over 100ml of the just-boiled water. Pour the rest of the water into a medium saucepan and stir in the stock cube until dissolved. Leave the mushrooms to soak.

Put the chicken breasts in the chicken stock – the liquid should just cover them. Place over a medium heat and bring to a gentle simmer, then cook for 10 minutes, turning after the first 5 minutes. The liquid should just simmer gently – don't let it boil. Lift the chicken breasts out of the stock with tongs and put them on a board to cool a little.

Place a large non-stick saucepan on the hob over a medium-high heat and add the oil. Fry the sliced chestnut mushrooms for 3 minutes until lightly browned, stirring constantly. Add the onion and garlic to the pan and cook with the mushrooms for 3 minutes until pale golden brown, stirring. Stir in the rice and cook for a minute with the vegetables, stirring constantly until the grains look translucent.

Reduce the heat to medium-low, add a large ladleful of the hot stock to the pan and stir well. As soon as it has been absorbed, add another ladleful. Continue gradually adding stock to the pan until it has all been used and the rice is looking swollen and creamy but isn't quite tender. This will take about 25 minutes and you need to keep stirring.

Just before the rice is ready, drain the dried mushrooms through a fine sieve placed over a bowl and reserve the soaking liquid. Roughly chop the mushrooms and add them to the pan with the rice. Stir in the mushroom soaking liquid and cook for a couple of minutes while you prepare the chicken. The risotto should look fairly saucy at this point, so if yours looks quite thick, stir in some extra water.

Cut the chicken into strips and stir them into the rice. Add the Parmesan and heat through for 2–3 minutes, then remove from the heat and check the seasoning. Stir in the crème fraiche, cover with a lid and leave the risotto to stand for 3–5 minutes before serving.

**SERVES 4**

10g dried wild mushrooms
1 litre just-boiled water
1 chicken stock cube
2 boneless, skinless chicken breasts
1 tbsp olive oil
150g small chestnut mushrooms, wiped and sliced
1 medium onion, finely chopped
2 garlic cloves, peeled and crushed
150g risotto rice (Arborio)
25g Parmesan cheese, finely grated
2 tbsp half-fat crème fraiche
flaked sea salt
freshly ground black pepper

*317 calories per portion*

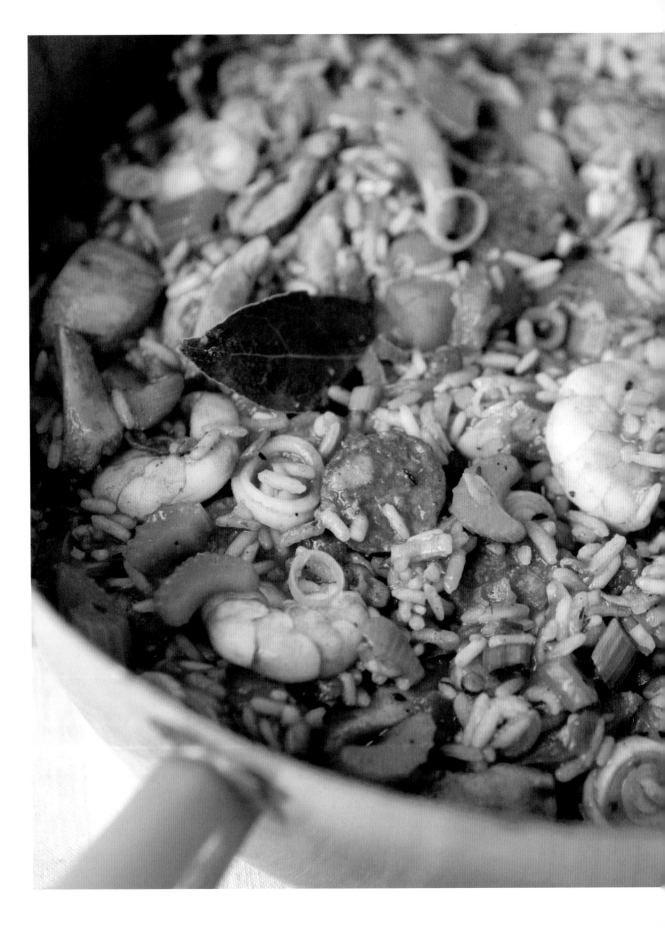

# SOUTHERN-STYLE JAMBALAYA

*Jambalaya is a wonderful rice dish that we got to know and love in Louisiana – a sort of Creole paella, really. This is our version, cutting down on the fat but keeping all the warm, spicy flavour.*

Cut the chicken thighs into bite-sized pieces, removing any excess fat, and season them with salt and pepper. Skin the sausage and cut it into 5mm slices. Heat the oil in a large non-stick frying pan or non-stick sauté pan and fry the chicken for 3 minutes over a medium heat until lightly coloured. Add the chorizo and cook for 30 seconds more, then transfer the chicken and chorizo with tongs to a large plate or tray.

Tip most of the oil out of the frying pan and chuck it away. Return the empty pan to the heat and turn the heat down to low. Stir in the onion, celery and green peppers and cook for 8–10 minutes until well softened, stirring occasionally.

Meanwhile, skin the tomatoes – see our top tip. Cut them in half and remove the green stem ends, then roughly chop the rest of the flesh – no need to deseed.

Stir the crushed garlic, paprika, cayenne, thyme, oregano and bay leaves into the frying pan and cook for 20–30 seconds, stirring. Increase the heat and add the chopped tomatoes and any juice that has collected on the board. Cook for 5 minutes or until the tomatoes are well softened, stirring regularly.

Return the chicken and chorizo to the pan, add the rice and cook for about a minute, stirring. Pour over the stock, season with a pinch of salt and lots of black pepper. Bring to a simmer and cook for about 10 minutes or until the rice is just tender and most of the liquid has evaporated or been absorbed by the rice, stirring occasionally. The rice should still be pretty saucy at this point, so if your rice takes longer to cook, you may need to add a little more stock.

Stir in the prawns and spring onions and cook for about 2 minutes more or until the prawns are hot, stirring regularly, then serve.

## SERVES 6

6 boneless, skinless chicken thighs
100g chorizo (we like picante)
1 tbsp olive oil
1 large onion, roughly chopped
4 slender celery sticks, cut into 1cm slices
2 small green peppers, deseeded and cut into 2cm chunks
5 large ripe vine tomatoes (about 475g)
3 garlic cloves, peeled and crushed
1 tbsp paprika
¼ tsp cayenne pepper
1 tsp dried thyme
1 tsp dried oregano
2 bay leaves
200g long-grain rice (we often use the easy-cook version)
450ml chicken stock, made with 1 chicken stock cube
100g cooked peeled king prawns, thawed if frozen
6 spring onions, sliced (including lots of green)
flaked sea salt
freshly ground black pepper

*341 calories per portion*

**Top tip:** *To skin tomatoes, make a small cross in the base of each tomato with the tip of a knife. Put the tomatoes in a heatproof bowl and cover with just-boiled water. Leave the tomatoes to stand for 30–60 seconds until the skins begin to wrinkle back, then drain. When the tomatoes are cool enough to handle, strip off the skins and chuck them away.*

# ITALIAN MEATBALLS
# WITH CHUNKY TOMATO SAUCE

*Lean minced pork can be the dieter's friend, but do check the fat content on the pack. You can make these with beef mince if you like, or a mixture of the two.*

**SERVES 4**

500g lean pork or beef mince (less than 10% fat) or 250g of each
½ medium onion, finely chopped
1 medium carrot, peeled and finely grated
2 garlic cloves, peeled and crushed
1 tsp dried oregano
½ tsp fine sea salt
1 tsp sunflower oil
freshly ground black pepper

**Tomato sauce**
2 tsp sunflower oil
½ medium onion, finely chopped
1 garlic clove, peeled and crushed
400g can of chopped tomatoes
100ml red wine or water
200ml cold water

*282 calories per portion*

To make the meatballs, put the mince in a large bowl and add the onion, carrot, garlic, oregano, salt and lots of freshly ground black pepper. Mix with clean hands until everything is well combined, then shape the mixture into 24 small balls; they should be slightly smaller than a walnut in its shell.

Pour the oil in a large non-stick frying pan or sauté pan and fry the meatballs over a medium heat for 5 minutes. Keep turning and rolling the meatballs around the pan until lightly browned, then transfer them to a plate.

To make the sauce, pour the sunflower oil into a medium non-stick saucepan and add the onion. Fry for 4 minutes, stirring regularly, then add the garlic and fry for 1 minute more.

Tip the tomatoes, red wine and water into the pan and bring to a gentle simmer. Cook for 5 minutes, stirring regularly. Add the browned meatballs to the sauce and bring back to a simmer.

Cover the pan loosely with a lid and leave the meatballs to simmer gently in the sauce for 20 minutes, stirring occasionally. After 20 minutes, remove the lid and continue simmering gently for another 15–20 minutes or until the sauce is thick. Stir often and add a little extra water if the sauce reduces too quickly. Serve hot with a small portion of pasta or lots of freshly cooked vegetables.

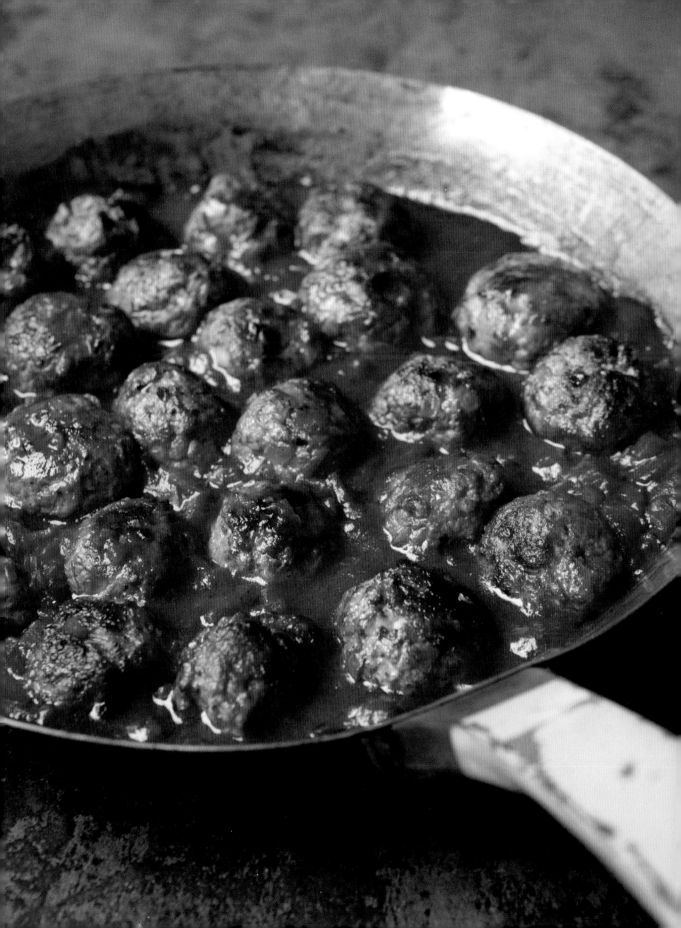

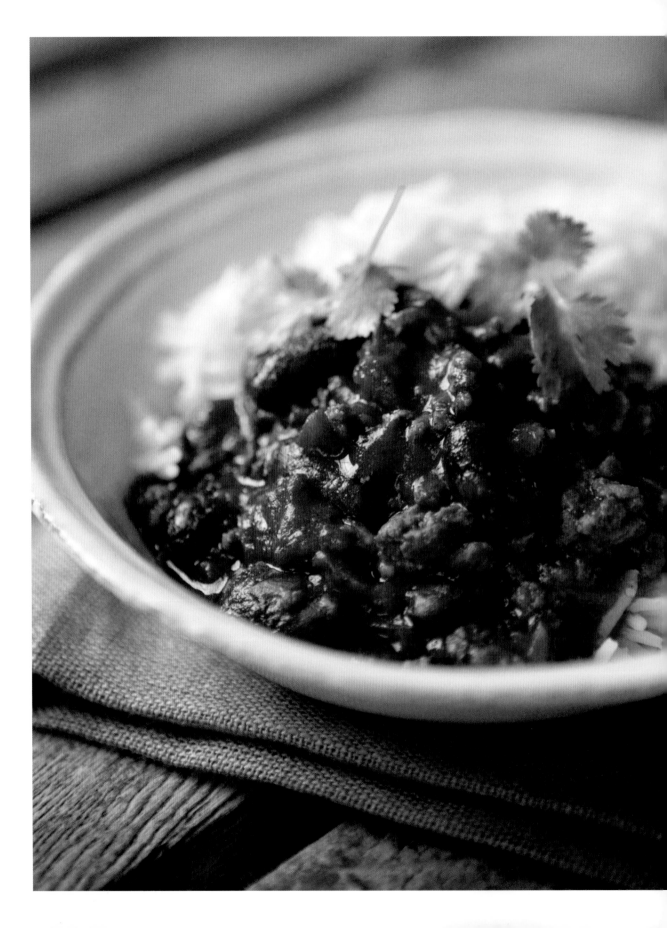

# CHILLI CON CARNE

*Here's a spicy classic you can still eat while on a diet. Serve with a salad and/or a very small portion of rice. Don't forget you've already got some carbs in the beans.*

Place a large non-stick saucepan over a medium heat and add the beef and onions. Cook together for 5 minutes, stirring the beef and squishing it against the sides of the pan to break up the lumps. Add the garlic, 1–2 teaspoons of chilli powder, depending on how hot you like your chilli, and the cumin and coriander. Fry together for 1–2 minutes more. Sprinkle over the flour and stir well.

Slowly add the wine and then the stock, stirring constantly. Tip the tomatoes and kidney beans into the pan and stir in the tomato purée, caster sugar, oregano and bay leaf. Season with a pinch of salt and plenty of freshly ground black pepper.

Bring to a simmer on the hob, then cover loosely with a lid. Reduce the heat and leave to simmer gently for 45 minutes, stirring occasionally until the mince is tender and the sauce is thick. Adjust the seasoning to taste and serve.

## SERVES 5

500g lean minced beef (10% or less fat)
2 medium onions, chopped
3 garlic cloves, peeled and finely chopped
1–2 tsp hot chilli powder
2 tsp ground cumin
2 tsp ground coriander
2 tbsp plain flour
150ml red wine or extra stock
300ml beef stock, made with 1 beef stock cube
400g can of chopped tomatoes
400g can of red kidney beans, drained and rinsed
3 tbsp tomato purée
1 tsp caster sugar
1 tsp dried oregano
1 bay leaf
flaked sea salt
freshly ground black pepper

*302 calories per portion (without rice)*

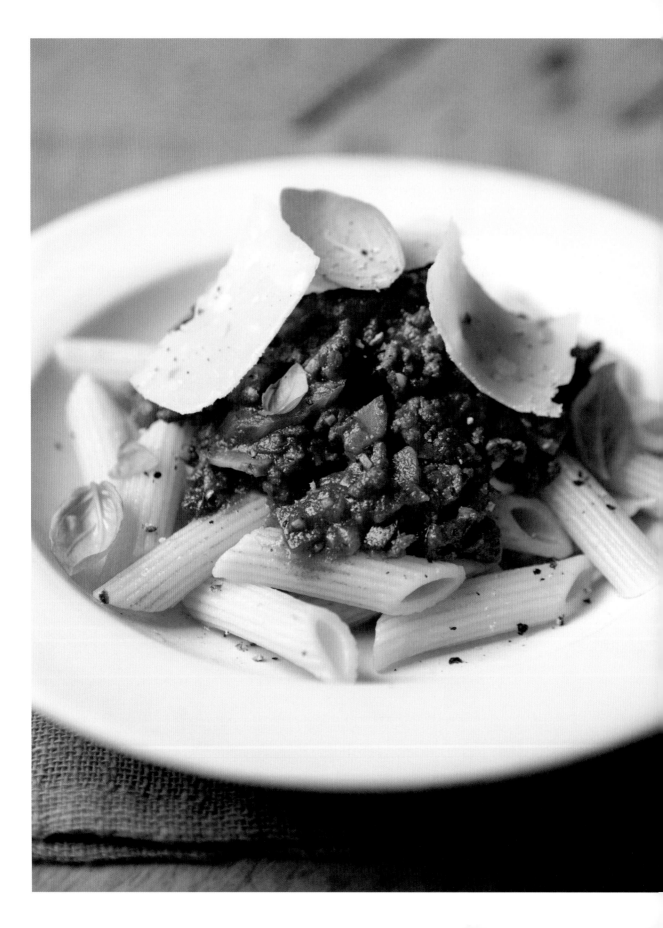

# RICH AND MEATY BOLOGNESE

*It sounds a bit mad but if you really want to go low-cal, serve your sauce on a pile of lightly boiled shredded cabbage. We won't say you can't tell the difference but it works. If you stick with the pasta, make sure to cook just 50 grams of pasta for each of the calorie counters.*

Place a large non-stick saucepan or flameproof casserole dish over a medium heat. Add the mince with the onions, garlic, celery, courgette and mushrooms and cook for 10 minutes until lightly coloured. Use a couple of wooden spoons to break up the meat as it cooks.

Stir in the wine, tomatoes, tomato purée, beef stock, oregano, dried chilli, if using, and bay leaves. Season with a good pinch of salt and plenty of freshly ground black pepper. Bring to the boil, then reduce the heat, cover loosely and simmer the sauce gently for 30 minutes, stirring occasionally.

Remove the lid and cook for a further 20–30 minutes uncovered until the mince is tender and the sauce is thick. Don't forget to stir, especially towards the end of the cooking time when the sauce will be getting thicker.

Mix the cornflour with the cold water to make a thin paste. Stir into the Bolognese and cook for another 1–2 minutes, stirring. Adjust the seasoning to taste and serve with a small portion of pasta (about 50g uncooked). Alternatively, if you want to go the cabbage route, lightly boil some finely shredded white cabbage and serve with the sauce. Add a few shavings of Parmesan cheese if you like, but don't forget that every bit adds calories.

**SERVES 6**

400g lean minced beef
2 medium onions, chopped
3 garlic cloves, finely chopped
1 celery stick, finely sliced
1 medium courgette, diced
175g small chestnut
mushrooms, wiped and sliced
150ml red wine or extra stock
400g can of chopped tomatoes
2 tbsp tomato purée
500ml beef stock, made with
1 beef stock cube
1 heaped tsp dried oregano
1 tsp dried chilli flakes (optional)
2 bay leaves
1 tbsp cornflour
1 tbsp cold water
flaked sea salt
freshly ground black pepper

*175 calories per portion*
*(without pasta)*

# SI AND DAVE'S WEIGHT-LOSS TIPS

———

We've come up with some sweet treats for you to enjoy once in a while. Don't overdo it though or you will slow down your weight loss.

———

Make cakes with sunflower oil instead of butter – see our carrot cake on page 156. We've found this helps make moister cakes with less fat. They keep well too.

———

Use reduced-sugar jam instead of the usual jams.

———

Fresh home-made jellies look really special and are easy to make. Kids of all ages love them.

———

Fresh fruit makes a good pud or snack, but remember that the swing it causes in your blood sugar levels can leave you feeling hungry. Just one apple or banana, or a couple of plums or satsumas, or perhaps a small bunch of grapes is all you should be eating at the moment. Still better than a choc bar though.

———

# PUDDINGS
# & CAKES

"The less sugar you eat the less
you want. I know this is true,
but it's hard sometimes."

*Dave*

# MOIST CARROT AND SULTANA CAKE

*We all know you can't be eating cake every day when you're keen to shed a few pounds, but a little of what you fancy can't be all bad. This cake is made with oil instead of butter and is super-moist, so non-dieters will love it too – if you let them have any.*

**SERVES 10**

3 medium carrots (about 250g total unpeeled weight)
3 large eggs
100ml sunflower oil, plus extra for greasing
100g soft light brown sugar
200g self-raising flour
100g sultanas
finely grated zest of ½ large well-scrubbed orange
1 tsp ground cinnamon
½ tsp grated nutmeg
1½ tsp baking powder

**Decoration**
2 tsp icing sugar
finely pared or grated zest of ½ well-scrubbed orange

*239 calories per slice*

Preheat the oven to 190°C/Fan 170°C/Gas 5. Grease a 23cm round loose-based cake tin with a little oil and line the base with baking parchment. Peel the carrots and grate them with a medium-fine grater – you should have about 200g of grated carrot.

Beat the eggs in a large bowl with a large metal whisk. Add the sunflower oil and sugar and whisk until well combined. Stir in the grated carrot, then add the flour, sultanas, orange zest, spices and baking powder. Stir together until just combined. Pour into the prepared cake tin and smooth the surface.

Bake in the centre of the oven for 25–30 minutes or until the cake is well risen and feels springy to the touch. It should be just beginning to shrink back from the sides of the tin. Leave to cool in the tin for 5 minutes then turn out and remove the lining paper. Leave to cool fully on a wire rack then transfer to a serving plate.

Sift the icing sugar over the cake and scatter grated or pared orange zest on top. This cake will keep well in the fridge for up to 3 days.

**Top tip:** *For a special occasion, you could add a cream cheese topping to this cake. Simply spread the cake with a 200g tub of light (medium-fat) soft cheese. Sprinkle with the grated orange zest and finish with sifted icing sugar. Don't forget that you'll be adding a few extra calories with the topping.*

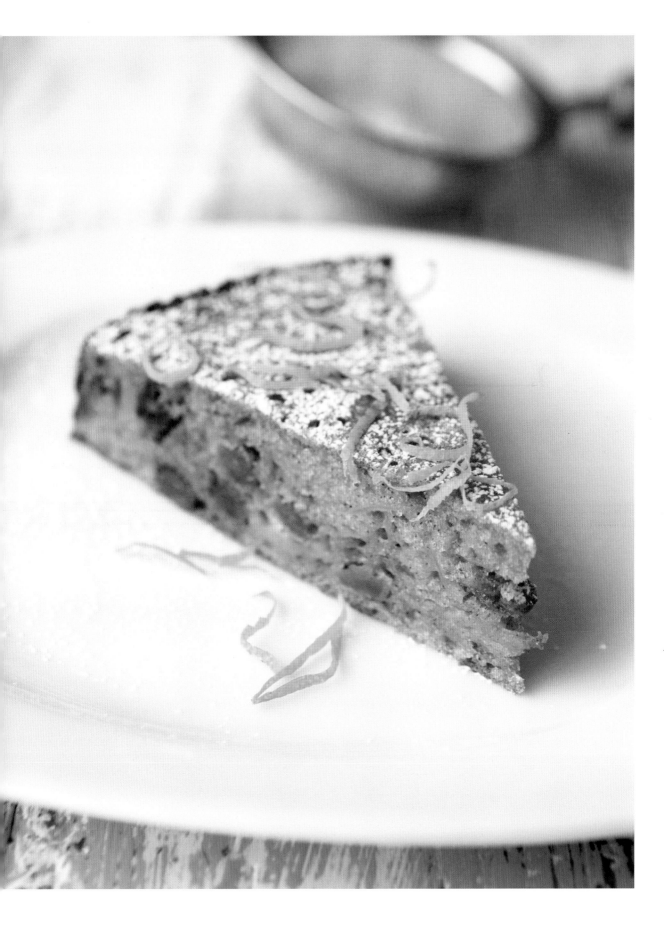

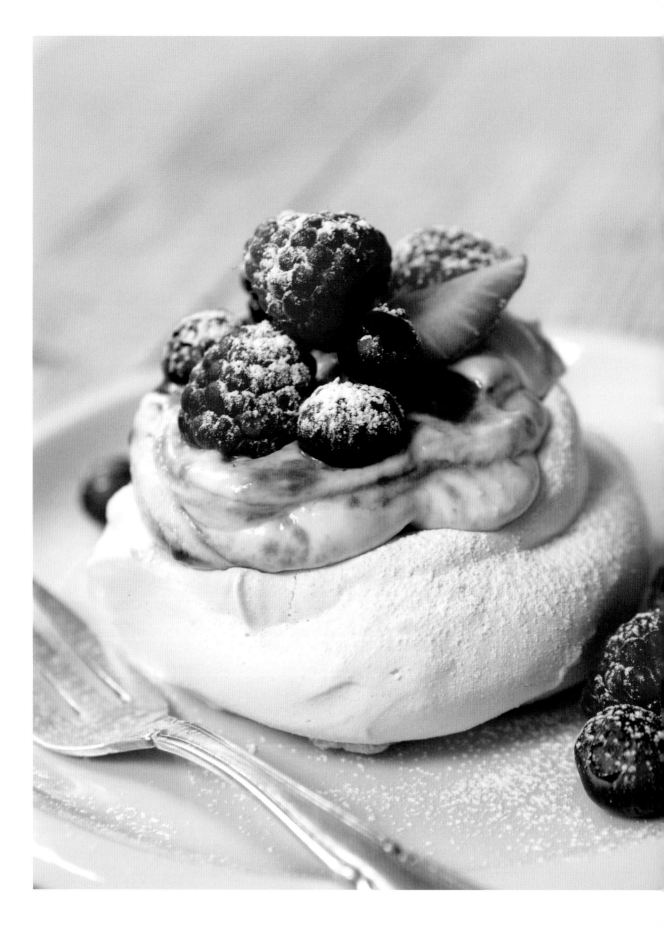

# SUMMER FRUIT MERINGUES

*Now these really are a treat! A perfect pud for that special Sunday lunch when you might allow yourself a few extra calories – and you can make up for it the next day.*

Preheat the oven to 150°C/Fan 130°C/Gas 2. Cut a piece of baking parchment large enough to line a large baking tray. Using a cookie cutter or small saucer to draw around and a dark pencil, mark out 6 circles, each measuring 9cm across, on the paper. Brush the baking sheet with a little sunflower oil and place the parchment on it, turning it over so the pencil marks are on the underside but still visible.

To make the meringue, put the egg whites in a large bowl and whisk with an electric whisk until they are stiff but not dry. They are ready when you can turn the bowl upside down without the egg whites sliding out.

Gradually whisk in the sugar, a tablespoon at a time, whisking for a few seconds in between each addition. Finally whisk in the vanilla extract and the cornflour until well combined. Using 2 pudding spoons, spoon the meringue on to the circles in billowing ring shapes, leaving a wide gap in the centre of each nest.

Reduce the oven temperature to 120°C/Fan 100°C/Gas ½. Place the tray of meringues in the oven and bake for 2 hours until dry. Turn the oven down more if they begin to colour. At the end of the cooking time, turn the oven off and leave the meringues to cool in the oven for several hours.

Put a meringue on each plate, handling them very carefully. Whip the cream and jam together in a large bowl with an electric whisk until the mixture forms soft peaks. Don't over-whip or it will separate. Stir in the crème fraiche.

Arrange a few strawberry halves in each meringue to fill the holes loosely. Spoon the raspberry cream on top, then add the rest of the fruit, dotting it on randomly. Dust with sifted icing sugar and serve.

## SERVES 6

**Meringues**
3 large egg whites
150g caster sugar
½ tsp pure vanilla extract
2 tsp cornflour
1 tsp sunflower oil

**Filling**
100ml double cream
25g seedless reduced-sugar raspberry jam
50g half-fat crème fraiche
200g small strawberries, hulled and halved
100g blueberries and/or blackberries
100g raspberries
1 tsp icing sugar, sifted, to decorate

*242 calories per portion*

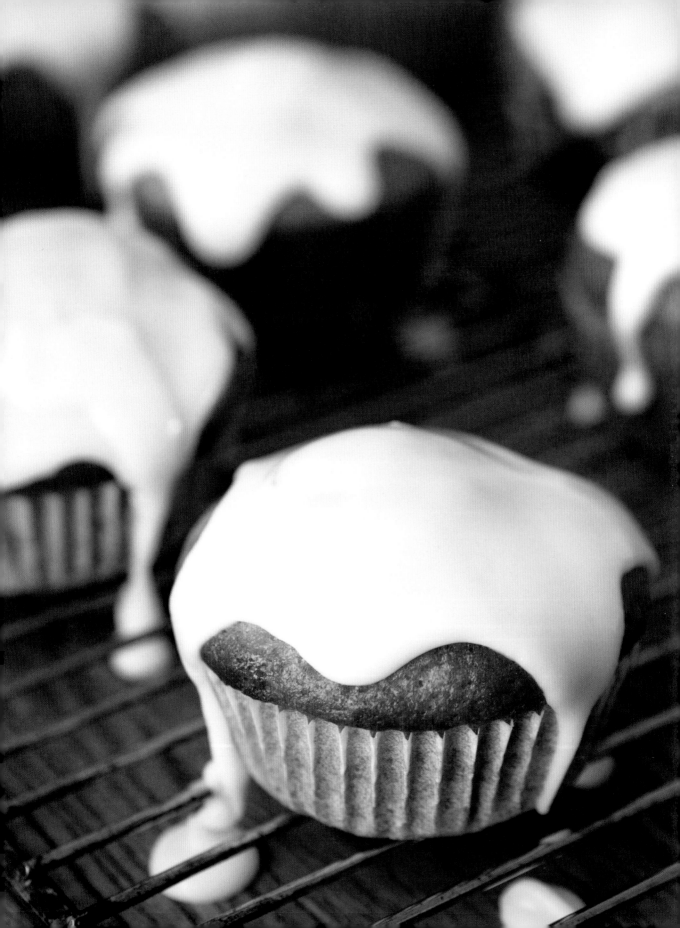

# SKINNY LEMON CUPCAKES WITH DRIZZLY ICING

*Cupcakes are all the rage but they can make you fat. Don't miss out on all the fun, give these low-cal versions a whirl. Just eat one mind, not the whole batch.*

Preheat the oven to 200°C/Fan 180°C/Gas 6. Line a 12-hole deep muffin tin with some non-stick paper cases or folded squares of baking parchment.

Sift the flour and bicarbonate of soda into a large bowl and stir in the sugar, blueberries and lemon zest. Make a well in the centre.

Beat the eggs with a large whisk until smooth, then beat in the yoghurt, milk and oil until well combined. Stir into the flour mixture with a large metal spoon until very lightly mixed.

Working quickly, divide the batter between the paper cases. Bake in the centre of the oven for 16–18 minutes or until the cupcakes are well risen and golden brown. Transfer them to a wire rack and leave to cool.

To make the lemon icing, mix the icing sugar and lemon juice in a small bowl until smooth and runny. Using a spoon, drizzle the icing over the cupcakes and leave to set for at least 30 minutes before serving.

## MAKES 12

200g self-raising flour
1 tsp bicarbonate of soda
75g golden caster sugar
100g blueberries
finely grated zest of 1 unwaxed lemon
2 large eggs
150ml low-fat natural yoghurt
2 tbsp semi-skimmed milk
50ml sunflower oil

### Lemon icing
100g icing sugar
4–4½ tsp fresh lemon juice

*167 calories per cupcake*

*Top tip:* *You can make these skinny cupcakes with plain dark chocolate instead of blueberries if you like. Use 100g of roughly chopped dark chocolate or drops or buttons and you will add about 43 calories to each cupcake. You can also flavour the cakes with ½ tsp of vanilla extract instead of lemon zest and use water instead of lemon juice to make the icing.*

# SWISS ROLL

*The only fat this cake contains is in the eggs – there is no added butter or oil – so you really can have your cake and eat it. There is quite a bit of sugar though, so don't go mad. Lovely for an occasional treat with a nice hot cup of tea.*

**SERVES 8**

butter, for greasing
3 large eggs
100g caster sugar, plus 1 tbsp
1 tsp vanilla extract
115g plain flour
150g seedless reduced-sugar raspberry jam, well stirred

*159 calories per slice*

Grease the base and sides of a 33 x 23cm Swiss roll tin and line it with baking parchment. Preheat the oven to 200°C/Fan 180°C/Gas 6. Put the eggs, sugar and vanilla in a heatproof bowl and place the bowl over a pan of gently simmering water. Whisk with an electric whisk until the mixture is pale, creamy and thick enough to leave a trail when you lift the whisk.

Carefully remove the bowl from the heat and whisk for a further 5 minutes. Sift over half the flour and, using a large metal spoon, lightly fold the flour into the egg mixture. Sift over the remaining flour and fold it in. It's important to use gentle movements to keep as much air as possible in the batter but watch out for pockets of flour.

Pour the mixture into the prepared tin and gently spread it with a spatula, so the base of the tin is evenly covered. Bake for 10 minutes until well risen, pale golden brown and firm to the touch. If you touch the centre of the sponge it should spring back immediately. Make sure the cake isn't overcooked or it won't roll.

While the sponge is cooking, place a damp tea towel on the work surface and cover with a sheet of baking parchment. Dredge with the tablespoon of sugar – this will help stop the sponge sticking. Working quickly, turn the cake out on to the sugared paper and carefully remove the baking parchment from the sponge. Make sure a long side of the cake is facing you.

Using a sharp knife, cut off thin strips of the crusty edges from the 2 long sides. Score the sponge lightly with a sharp knife from top to bottom about 2.5cm in from the left-hand side. It will look a bit like a margin on the side of a page. This will help make a nice tight turn when you start to roll the sponge but make sure you only go a little less than halfway through.

Spread the sponge all over with the jam. Roll the Swiss roll from the scored end, starting with the tight turn to make a good round shape. Leave the cake to cool on a wire rack, then place it on a serving plate or board. Cut into slices to serve.

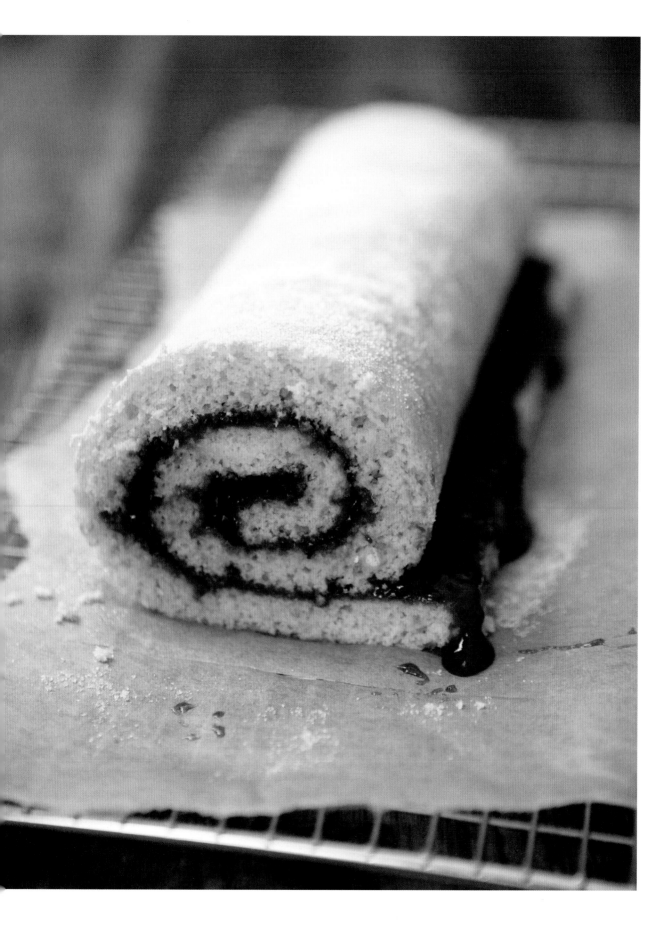

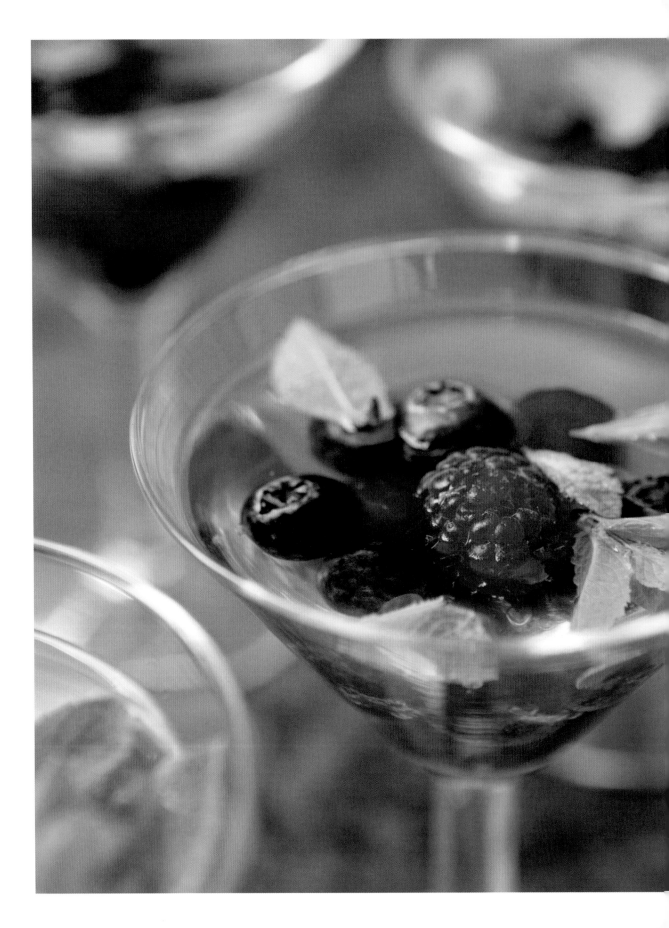

# SPARKLING LEMONADE AND LIME JELLY

*We all feel like something sweet from time to time and this sparkly fruity jelly is as low in calories as it gets. Keep some in the fridge as little life-savers for those moments of temptation.*

Put the gelatine sheets in a medium bowl and cover them with cold water. Leave to soak for 5 minutes or until they become very soft and floppy. Turn the gelatine sheets a couple of times to make sure they don't stick together in a clump.

Pour the lime or lemon squash and water into a small saucepan and heat very gently for a few seconds until just warm. Remove from the heat. Take the gelatine sheets in your hands and squeeze them over the bowl to remove any excess water.

Plop the gelatine into the pan with the squash and stir well until it melts into the liquid. If it doesn't melt almost immediately, return the pan to the heat and warm through gently, stirring constantly until the liquid is smooth and clear.

Pour the diet lemonade into a large measuring jug. Add the gelatine mixture, stirring constantly with a long-handled spoon until it is thoroughly combined. Pour it slowly as the lemonade will froth up.

Drop the berries into 6 wine glasses or tumblers, then pour almost all the jelly mixture gently over the top – keep back about 100ml of the lemonade jelly. Place the glasses on a tray and cover with clingfilm. Carry them carefully to the fridge and leave for 4 hours or until lightly set. Leave the reserved jelly at room temperature and do not allow it to set.

Take the jellies out of the fridge, and add a few mint leaves to each jelly if you like. Stir each jelly a couple of times with a fork to create bubbles of air, but be careful not to mash the fruit. Pour the runny reserved jelly over the top to create a smooth surface for each dessert. Cover with cling film and return to the fridge for a further 2–3 hours or until set.

**SERVES 6**

6 sheets of leaf gelatine (about 10g)
4 tbsp lime or lemon squash (with no added sugar)
50ml water
600ml diet lemonade
100g fresh raspberries
100g fresh blueberries
small handful of fresh mint leaves (optional)

*20 calories per portion*

*Top tip:* *If you are short of time, don't keep back some of the jelly, use it all at once. The jellies won't look as bubbly but they will still taste great.*

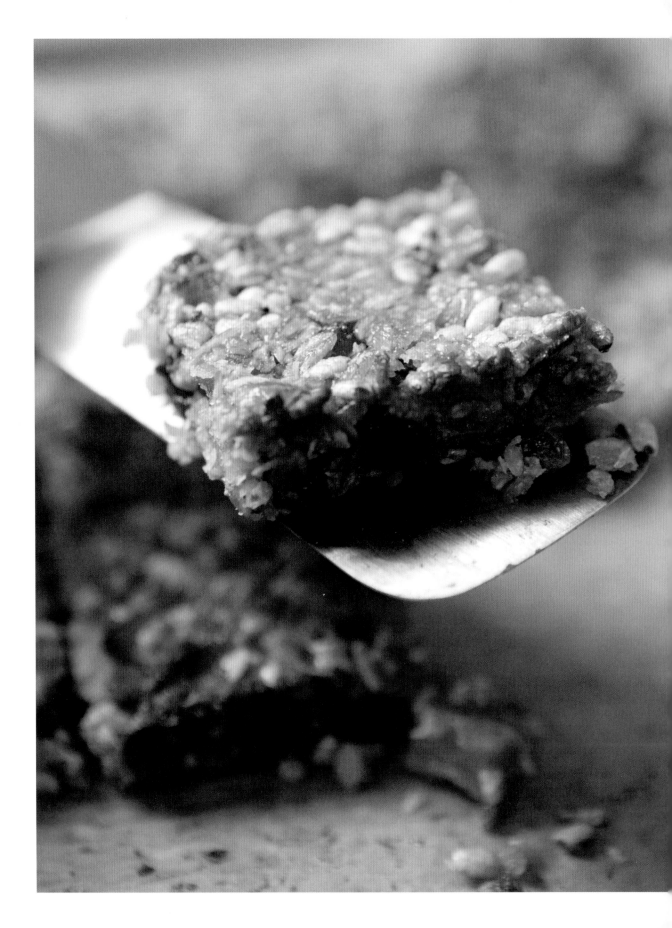

# CHEWY CRANBERRY AND APRICOT BITES

*These little goodies are sweetened with maple syrup and have a lovely soft, chewy texture. Great for an occasional treat or to pop into lunch boxes, but go easy as the dried fruit means they aren't totally low in calories.*

Preheat the oven to 190°C/Fan 170°C/Gas 5. Line a 20 x 30cm brownie tin with baking parchment. Scatter the almonds over a baking tray and bake in the oven for 5–6 minutes or until lightly toasted, then tip them into a large mixing bowl. Cut the apricots into small pieces and add them to the bowl along with the cranberries, sultanas, rice cereal and coconut.

Put the maple syrup and apple juice in a large saucepan and warm over a low heat, stirring once or twice. Add the oats and bring to a gentle simmer, stirring. Cook for 3–4 minutes, stirring constantly until the oats become thick and porridgy – keep a close eye on it as the mixture does get very sticky. Remove the pan from the heat and stir in all the other ingredients until thoroughly mixed.

Spoon the mixture into the prepared tin and flatten the surface with a spatula to press everything down well. Pop into the preheated oven and bake for 40–45 minutes until the mixture is golden brown and the surface is crisp. Take out of the oven and press once more with a spatula – this will make the bites easier to cut later. Leave to cool in the tin for about 30 minutes before cutting into small squares with a sharp knife.

Transfer to a board and lift the squares off the lining paper. Store in an airtight container lined with baking parchment for up to 5 days.

**MAKES 24**

25g flaked almonds
40g no-soak dried apricots
40g dried cranberries
40g sultanas
75g unsweetened puffed rice cereal
40g desiccated coconut
150ml maple syrup
400ml apple juice (preferably the cloudy type)
125g porridge oats

*82 calories per piece*

# PLUM RICE PUDDING

*Those little pots of rice pudding you can buy in supermarkets make a nice sweet treat, but they are expensive and they contain lots of sugar. It's so much cheaper to make your own and really easy. Eat the rice pudding on its own or topped with a fruity compote. We like plums, but use any lightly stewed fruit you like – apples, pears and summer berries all work well.*

**SERVES 4**

100g pudding rice
400ml semi-skimmed milk
200ml cold water
¼ tsp vanilla extract
1 tsp caster sugar (preferably golden)

**Compote**
3 ripe plums, stoned and quartered
6 tbsp cold water
1 tsp caster sugar (preferably golden)

*134 calories per portion*
*(with compote)*

Put the rice, milk, water and vanilla extract in a medium non-stick saucepan and bring to a gentle simmer over a medium heat. Cook for 16–18 minutes or until the rice is tender and the sauce is creamy, stirring regularly. Don't forget that it will continue to thicken as it cools, so add a little extra water if serving cold. Stir frequently towards the end of the cooking time as the mixture will be thickening up. Sweeten with a little caster sugar and serve warm or chilled with or without the topping.

To make the compote topping, put the plums, water and sugar in a saucepan and bring to a gentle simmer. Cook for 5 minutes, stirring gently, until the plums are softened but still holding their shape. Add a little extra water if you need.

Spoon the rice pudding into tumblers or dessert dishes and top with the plum compote. Delicious warm or cold.

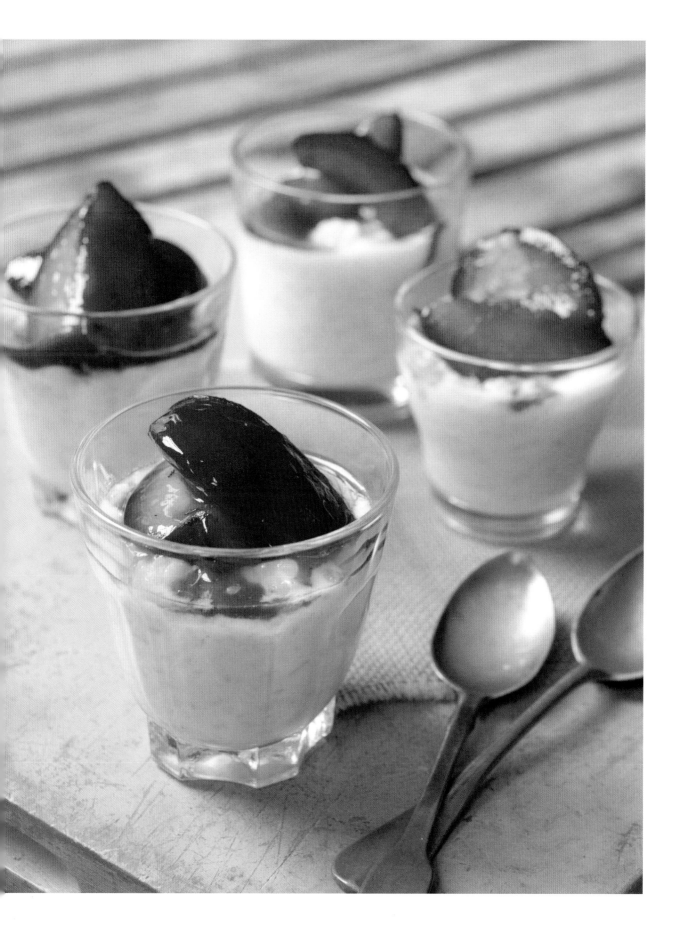

# SI AND DAVE'S WEIGHT-LOSS TIPS

———

Taking your own lunch to work helps you keep control of your calorie intake. Shop-bought sandwiches are often surprisingly high in calories and those little pots of salad can be drenched in dressing, so high in fat.

———

Make a big batch of soup so you can take some to work to heat up and enjoy with a crispbread or two. It keeps well in the fridge for several days. A mug of soup makes a good snack too.

———

Pack your lunch box with the ingredients for a topless sandwich (see page 177) and put it all together when you're ready. That way, your topless sarnie doesn't get a soggy bottom.

———

A home-made pasta or rice salad makes an ideal take-to-work lunch to eat with some extra veg, such as strips of pepper or carrot sticks.

———

Guard against temptation by keeping a good selection of healthy snacks, such as crispbreads, olives and rice cakes.

———

If you're hungry between meals, drink lots of water. It has no calories and will help you feel full.

———

# LUNCH BOXES
# & SNACKS

"The best way to avoid the bad
stuff is to keep plenty of the
good stuff to hand."

*Si*

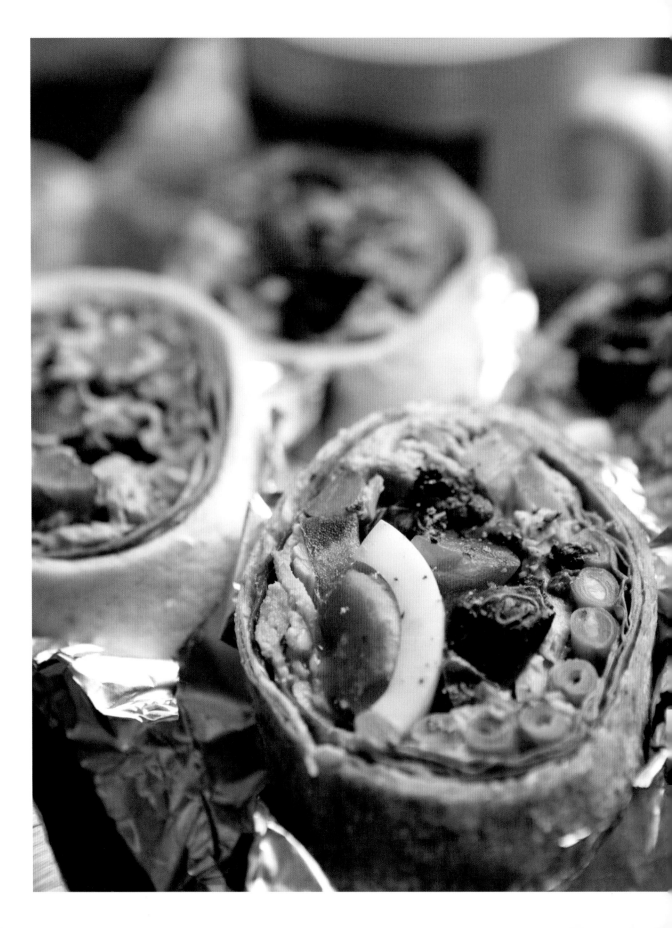

# TUNA NIÇOISE WRAP

*We made these protein-packed wraps to take on a picnic and they were substantial and tasty – a feast in a flatbread. They survived the journey in a bicycle pannier well too, so just the thing for a day out in the hills and dales.*

Bring a pan of water to the boil, add the beans and cook for 4 minutes. Lift the beans out with a slotted spoon and dunk them into a large bowl of cold water. Alternatively, tip the beans into a sieve and rinse them under running water until cold. Drain.

To boil the egg, put the pan back on the heat, add the egg and bring the water back to the boil. Cook for 8 minutes, then put the egg in a sieve under running water until cold. Leave the egg in cold water while you prepare the rest of the filling.

Mix the mayonnaise, capers, gherkins, herbs and a few twists of ground black pepper in a bowl. Add the tuna and stir everything lightly, without mashing the tuna too much. Peel the egg, then slice it into quarters, lengthwise.

Place the tortillas on a board and cover each one with a layer of spinach leaves, leaving a gap of about 5cm at the top and bottom of the tortilla. Add the green beans, all heading in one direction. Divide the tuna mixture between the tortillas, then the egg and tomato pieces. Sprinkle with the olives, pressing each one lightly between your thumb and finger to flatten slightly.

Fold the top and bottom of each wrap inwards to cover most of the filling and then roll up fairly tightly. Wrap them in foil – no need do this if eating immediately – then chill until ready to eat. Eat within 24 hours and transport with an ice pack if serving as a packed lunch. Unwrap the foil as you eat the wrap.

## SERVES 2

50g green beans, trimmed
1 medium egg (fridge cold)
2 tbsp light mayonnaise
1 tbsp baby capers, drained
4 baby gherkins, drained and sliced
¼ tsp dried mixed herbs
185g can of tuna in spring water
2 large flour tortillas or wraps (white or wholemeal or a combination)
small handful of baby spinach leaves
1 large ripe tomato, cut into 8 pieces
20g pitted black olives in brine, drained
freshly ground black pepper

*325 calories per portion*

**Top tip:** *If you are taking your wrap to work, don't forget to use a cool bag and ice pack to keep it chilled and in tip-top condition until you are ready to eat.*

# SIMPLE TUNA AND SWEETCORN PASTA SALAD

*This makes a really satisfying lunch and it's easy to take to work with you in a plastic box. It's low in calories too, as long as you're careful with the dressing. Try our trick of diluting the mayo with some water – works a treat.*

**SERVES 4**

100g pasta shapes, such as fusilli or penne
200g can of tuna in spring water, drained
195g can of sweetcorn, drained
3 tbsp light mayonnaise
3 tbsp cold water
2 tsp white wine vinegar
10 cherry tomatoes, halved (about 100g)
¼ cucumber, cut into rough 1.5cm dice
1 yellow pepper, deseeded and cut into rough 1.5cm dice
2 spring onions, finely sliced
freshly ground black pepper
romaine or little gem lettuce leaves, to serve (optional)

*183 calories per portion*

Half fill a large saucepan with cold water and bring to the boil. Add the pasta, stir well and bring the water back to the boil. Cook for 8–10 minutes until tender, or according to the packet instructions, stirring occasionally.

Rinse the pasta in a colander under running water until cold, then drain well and tip it into a large mixing bowl. Flake the tuna on to the pasta with a fork and scatter the sweetcorn on top.

Put the mayonnaise, water and vinegar in a small bowl and whisk with a small metal whisk until smooth. Pour the mixture over the pasta.

Add the tomatoes, cucumber, pepper and spring onions, season with a few twists of black pepper and toss all the ingredients lightly together. Serve with lettuce leaves if you like. Perfect for lunch boxes and picnics.

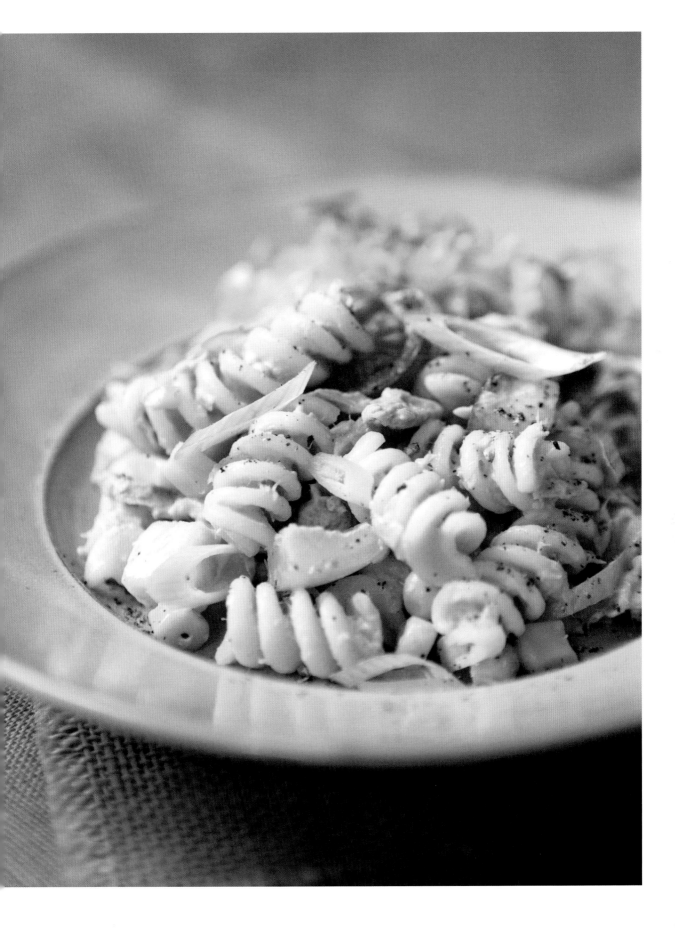

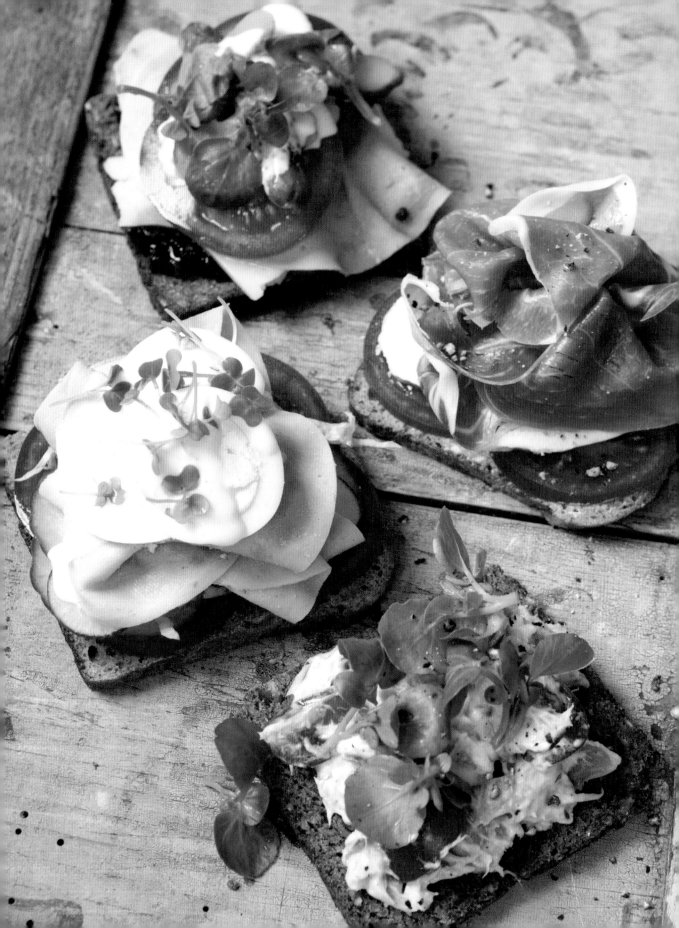

# TOPLESS SANDWICHES

*To reduce the calorie count but not the satisfaction factor of your sandwiches, try going topless: make your sandwiches with just one slice of bread and loads of filling. We've been enjoying dense rye pumpernickel-style bread, which takes a bit of getting used to but makes brilliant open-topped sandwiches. It contains no wheat and is very satisfying – and is slightly lower in calories than thick-sliced wholegrain bread. Try not to cut your bread too thick – that's cheating – and toast or griddle it if you like. If you want to take a topless sandwich as a packed lunch, take all the bits and bobs separately and put them together when you're ready to eat. Here are some of our favourites.*

## CHICKEN AND PARMA HAM

Spread a slice of rye bread with ½ teaspoon of softened butter. Top with a sliced tomato, then slice half a skinless roast chicken breast and arrange it over the tomato. Top with 2 slices of Parma ham. Toss some shredded lettuce and sliced cucumber and place alongside the bread. Mix 1 teaspoon of light mayonnaise with ½ teaspoon of fresh lemon juice and ½ teaspoon cold water until smooth and spoon over the salad. Season with black pepper.

*331 calories*

## MACKEREL PÂTÉ AND WATERCRESS

Skin a 55g smoked mackerel fillet and put the flesh in a bowl. Add a tablespoon of low-fat natural yoghurt and 1 teaspoon of light mayonnaise and mash roughly with a fork. Add 1 tablespoon of finely chopped red onion and 3 cherry tomatoes cut into quarters and mix lightly. Put a slice of rye bread on a plate and top with lots of fresh watercress leaves. Spoon the mackerel mixture over the watercress and season with black pepper.

*370 calories*

## A VERY ENGLISH SANDWICH

Put a slice of rye bread on a plate and top with a large sliced tomato and a few cucumber slices. Add some torn lettuce leaves and a few slices of radish. Top with 4 slices of wafer-thin ham (about 40g) and a sliced hard-boiled egg. Drizzle with 2 teaspoons of salad cream and snip over some salad cress.

*301 calories*

## CHEESE AND PICKLE

Put a slice of rye bread on a plate and spread with 1 teaspoon of farmhouse pickle or chutney. Top with 40g sliced half-fat mature Cheddar and 1 slice of lean ham. Add 1 sliced tomato and 2 sliced dill gherkins. Spoon over 1 teaspoon of salad cream and serve garnished with fresh watercress.

*288 calories*

# EGG, BACON AND ASPARAGUS FLAN

*A light tart that melts in the mouth, this feels like a real treat and it's a cinch to make. There's not even any rolling involved. If you like, leave the asparagus out of the filling mixture or add extra ingredients of your own. Sautéed mushrooms, blanched broccoli and roasted peppers all work well.*

**SERVES 6**

1 bunch of young asparagus, about 10 spears, trimmed
5 rashers of dry-cure smoked back bacon
1 tsp olive oil
1 medium onion, finely sliced
25g cornflour
300ml semi-skimmed milk
3 large eggs, beaten
25g extra-mature Cheddar cheese, finely grated
flaked sea salt
freshly ground black pepper

**Pastry**
1 tbsp sunflower oil, plus extra for oiling the tin
4 sheets of filo pastry, each about 32 x 38cm

*245 calories per portion*

Slice the asparagus into lengths of about 5cm. Half fill a large non-stick frying pan with water and bring to the boil. Add the asparagus, bring back to the boil and cook for 1 minute until just tender. Drain and rinse under running water until cold, then pat dry. Trim any fat off the bacon and cut it into 1cm strips. Return the pan to a low heat, add the oil and gently fry the onion and bacon until lightly browned, stirring regularly. Add the onion and bacon to the bowl with the asparagus, toss lightly and leave to cool. Preheat the oven to 200°C/Fan 180°C/Gas 6. Place a baking tray in the oven to heat.

Lightly oil a 20cm loose-based fluted flan tin that's about 3.5cm deep. Pour the rest of the oil into a small bowl. Place a sheet of filo pastry in the flan tin, pressing it firmly against the base and sides. Using the tip of a pastry brush, brush the pastry with a little oil then cover with a second pastry sheet at a right angle to the first. Brush with more oil and cover with a third sheet at the same angle to the first. Brush with the oil and cover with a fourth sheet, running in the same direction as the second. Roll and crumple the overhanging pastry back on to the rim of the tin, lifting slightly above it, and brush lightly with the remaining oil. Place the tin on the baking tray.

Put the cornflour in a non-stick saucepan and stir in 50ml of the milk to make a thin paste. Pour over 200ml of the milk and stir well. Bring to a simmer, stirring constantly. Cook for 1 minute over a medium heat, stirring, until the sauce is thick and smooth. Season, then remove from the heat and stir in the rest of the milk to cool and loosen the sauce. Stir in the beaten eggs until thoroughly combined.

Scatter half the asparagus, bacon and onion mixture over the base of the pastry case and pour the white sauce gently on top. Scatter the remaining asparagus and bacon mixture on top and press down lightly, then sprinkle evenly with the cheese. Bake on the preheated baking tray in the centre of the oven for 25–30 minutes or until the pastry is lightly browned and crisp and the filling is set. Take the flan out of the oven and leave to cool in the tin for 10 minutes before removing. Serve warm or cold.

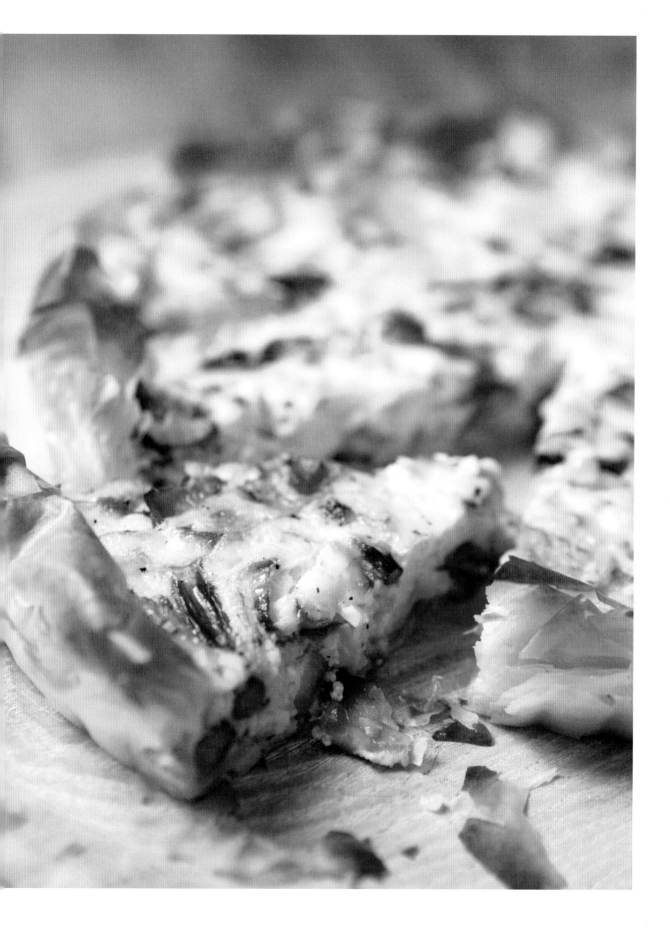

# CHEESE, LEEK AND ONION PASTIES

*You can't have a Hairy Biker book without a pasty so here they are. When only a pasty will do, we are here to rescue you with another hand-held lovely from our recipe vaults, this time with a special low-fat crust. Good for vegetarians too.*

**MAKES 8**

400g potatoes, preferably Maris Pipers, peeled and cut into rough 2cm chunks
300ml cold water
½ vegetable stock cube
350g leeks (2 medium), trimmed and cut into 5mm slices
1 medium onion, finely chopped
500g premium white bread mix
plain flour, for rolling
100g half-fat mature Cheddar, finely grated
1 tbsp semi-skimmed milk
freshly ground black pepper

*231 calories per portion*

Put the potatoes in a large non-stick saucepan and add the cold water. Crumble over the vegetable stock cube and set over a high heat. Bring to the boil and cook for 5 minutes. Add the leek and onion to the pan with the potato and stock and return to a fast simmer. Cook for another 8 minutes or until the vegetables are tender and all the liquid has evaporated. Stir regularly, especially towards the end of the cooking time so the potatoes don't stick. Remove the pan from the heat and set aside to cool.

To make the 'pastry' cases, make the bread dough by hand until smooth and elastic according to the packet instructions. Follow the directions up to the point at which the dough is shaped ready for baking. Because it is a bread dough, the 'pastry' won't feel as stiff as usual but it shouldn't be sticky so add a little extra plain flour if necessary. Roll the dough into 8 evenly sized balls.

Roll out each ball of dough on a lightly floured surface into a circle about 18cm across. Turn the dough every couple of rolls so you get a good even shape, but don't worry too much as they don't have to be perfect. Stir the grated cheese into the cooled potato mixture and season with lots of black pepper. Preheat the oven to 220°C/ Fan 200°C/Gas 7.

Spoon an eighth of the filling mixture on to one of the dough circles, placing it in a long heap down the centre and leaving a 2cm gap at each end. Lightly brush all around the edge of the dough with milk. Bring 2 sides up around the filling and press the edges together to seal firmly. Crimp the edges neatly.

Put the pasty on a baking tray lightly dusted with flour and make the rest in the same way. You'll need to use 2 baking trays or bake 1 batch after the other. Brush the pasties with more milk to glaze. Bake the pasties for 15 minutes, then cover them loosely with foil and bake for another 10–12 minutes or until lightly browned and hot inside. You may need to leave the lower tray in the oven for a few minutes longer than the one on the higher shelf. Serve warm or cold.

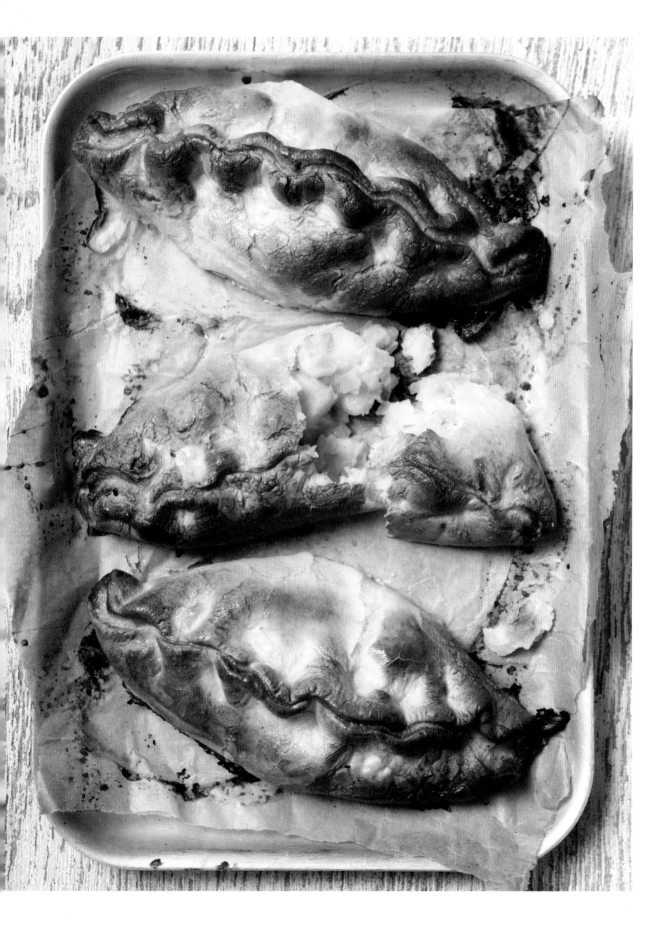

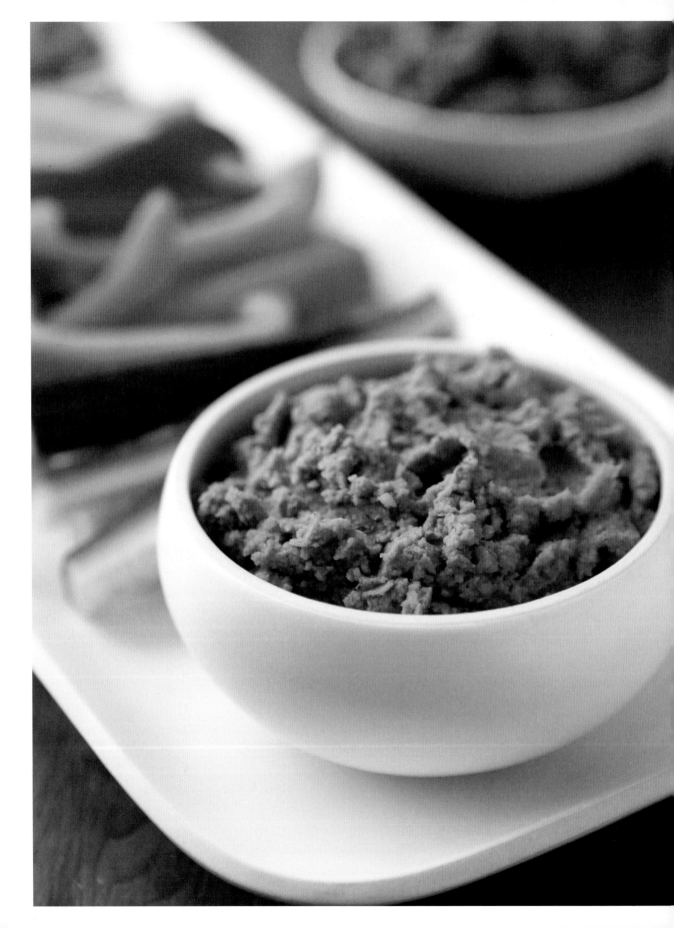

# ROASTED RED PEPPER HUMMUS

*This tasty dip makes a great snack with a few veg sticks. We like to have some of this in the fridge when the yearning for an in-between-meals mouthful gets too great.*

Preheat the grill to its hottest setting and line a grill pan or baking tray with foil. Cut the peppers in half lengthways, remove the stalks and deseed. Put the pepper halves, cut side down, on the lined tray.

Place the peppers on a shelf close to the heat and grill for 15 minutes or until the skins are blackened and charred. Remove the pan and leave the peppers for 10 minutes or until cool enough to handle.

Heat the olive oil in a small frying pan. Add the chopped onion, ground coriander and ground cumin. Fry over a medium heat for 3–4 minutes until softened, stirring occasionally, then leave to cool for 5 minutes.

Scoop the chopped onion mixture into the bowl of a food processor. Peel off the charred pepper skins and chuck them away. Tear the pepper flesh into pieces and add to the food processor with the onion. Then add the chickpeas, garlic, chilli, lemon zest and salt and blend until the mixture is as smooth as possible. You may need to remove the lid and push the mixture down once or twice with a spatula until you have the consistency you like. Leave it a bit chunkier if you like or make half the chickpeas very smooth and then add the rest for a final blitz.

Spoon the dip into a serving dish, or into small plastic containers if you want to take some for your lunch box, and eat with pieces of raw carrot, cucumber or other veg, or with dried vegetable crisps. Store it in the fridge and eat within 2 days.

**SERVES 6–8**

2 large red peppers
1 tbsp olive oil
½ small onion, finely chopped
1 heaped tsp ground coriander
1 heaped tsp ground cumin
400g can of chickpeas, drained and rinsed
2 garlic cloves, peeled and crushed
1 long red chilli, deseeded and roughly chopped
finely grated zest of ½ unwaxed lemon
1 tsp fine sea salt

*89 calories per portion (if serving 6)*
*67 calories per portion (if serving 8)*

# SNACKS

*If you're anything like us, you'll feel a bit peckish during the day between meals, but we've got into the habit of keeping some healthy low-cal snacks to hand so we don't head for the biscuit tin. Crispbreads are low in calories and can be topped with all sorts of ingredients, so we like to have a few different sorts as well as some rice or corn cakes in the cupboard. A tub of reduced-fat hummus is also a brilliant standby to enjoy with a few cut-up veggies for dipping. Be careful of your portion size though – no more than a couple of tablespoons for a snack. Avoid cheesy or creamy dips or you could be tempted to eat more calories than you need.*

*Most of these snacks are about 100 calories each, but the cheese and pickle has about 138.*

## PEANUT BUTTER AND APPLE

Spread 1 corn cake with 10g of peanut butter. Cut a quarter of an apple into slices, removing the core, and place on top of the peanut butter.

## MARINATED OLIVES

Marinated olives have lots of flavour. A 50g serving – about 8 olives – makes a great snack.

## HUMMUS AND VEGETABLES

Put 2 tablespoons of lemon and coriander hummus on a plate and serve with vegetable sticks.

## CHEESE AND PICKLE

Thinly slice 20g of half-fat Cheddar and place it on top of 2 oatcakes. Top each one with 1 teaspoon of farmhouse pickle.

## EMMENTAL AND TOMATOES

Cut 1 thin slice of Emmental cheese into strips and serve with cherry tomatoes or vegetable sticks.

## HAM AND PICKLE

Top 2 rye crispbreads with 4 slices of wafer-thin ham and 2 teaspoons of pickle.

## COTTAGE CHEESE AND TOMATO

Spread 30g of cottage cheese over 2 wholegrain rye crispbreads. Halve 3 cherry tomatoes and place them on top of the cottage cheese.

## ROAST CHICKEN, HAM AND GRAPES

Make up a small plate with about 50g of sliced skinless roast chicken breast, 1 slice of Parma ham and a 25g bunch of grapes.

## PRAWN AND CUCUMBER

Place slices of cucumber on a rye crispbread and top with 2 tablespoons of reduced-fat prawn cocktail. Season with a grinding of black pepper.

## SMOKED SALMON AND GHERKINS

Fold 2 slices of smoked salmon on to a plate and serve with 2–3 gherkins and cherry tomatoes.

## TROUT PÂTÉ

Place 30g of hot-smoked trout in a bowl with 1 tablespoon of low-fat yoghurt and mash together with a fork. Spread the trout mixture over 3 thin multigrain crispbread fingers. Thinly slice some cucumber and place on top of the trout.

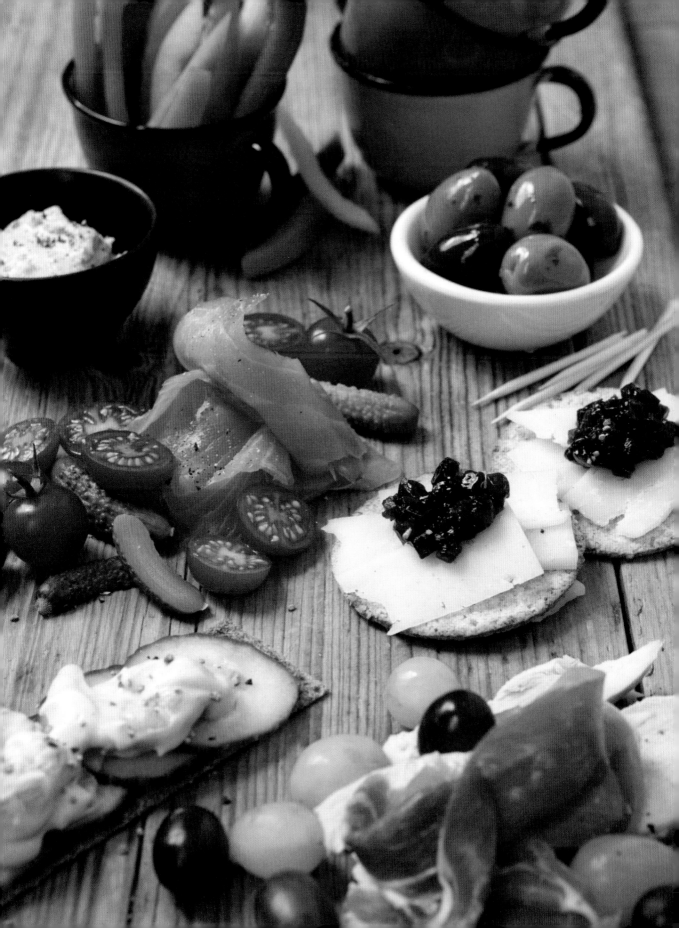

# MENUS FOR YOUR FIRST WEEK

We've put together these menu suggestions to get you started on your diet and give you an idea of what sort of meals you might have. You can be as flexible as you like; it's about making small changes to the way you cook – and eat – rather than getting stressed trying to squeeze your lifestyle into some one else's idea of healthy living. All our recipes have been carefully calorie counted, so you really can't go wrong. If you have extra calories one day, pick dishes with fewer for the next. It's about balancing your total calories for the week rather than worrying about each day.

Not everyone wants – or has time – to cook different things every day and you might prefer to make a big batch of soup or pasta salad at the start of the week and enjoy that for lunch over several days. Or you might like to finish up some leftovers from the day before for lunch or supper. We often make a big batch of stew, divide it into portions and pop it in the fridge, or freezer, to enjoy another day.

Allow yourself a couple of snacks every day, but make sure they're low in calories – check out our suggestions on page 184. Forget the crisps and other junk food. Drink tea and coffee as usual, but use semi-skimmed milk. Drink plenty of water, still or fizzy, and add a little no-sugar squash to encourage you to drink more of it. Try to keep alcohol to the weekend, if at all, and aim to drink just 1 or 2 glasses, no more. Again, get medical advice before starting a diet.

## MONDAY

*2 boiled eggs and 1 rye crispbread*
*Minestrone soup (page 33) and a topless sandwich of your choice (page 177)*
*Chilli con carne (page 151) with small portion of rice and salad*

## TUESDAY

*Cranberry and almond muesli with semi-skimmed milk (page 17)*
*Minted pea and feta omelette (page 31) with with a large mixed salad (page 111)*
*Salmon with chilli and ginger (page 48) with a small portion of rice and*
*stir-fried vegetables (from a pack)*

# WEDNESDAY

*Toasted crumpets with fruit (page 14)*
*Tuna and sweetcorn pasta salad (page 174)*
*Paprika chicken (page 91) with a small portion of rice and some green beans*

# THURSDAY

*2 scrambled eggs on 1 slice of wholegrain toast*
*Golden vegetable soup (page 35) and a topless sandwich of your choice (page 177)*
*Skinny beef lasagne (page 76) with with a large mixed salad (page 111)*

# FRIDAY

*Fresh fruit compote with home-made granola (page 23)*
*Tuna niçoise wrap (page 173)*
*Southern-style jambalaya (page 147) with green salad*

# SATURDAY

*Bacon with tomatoes and poached eggs (page 19)*
*Chicken caesar salad (page 105)*
*Mediterranean beefburgers (page 53) with a large mixed salad (page 111)*

# SUNDAY

*Scrambled eggs with smoked salmon (page 20)*
*Lemon and thyme roasted chicken with new potatoes and fresh vegetables (page 62),*
*followed by summer fruit meringues (page 159)*
*2 slices of ham with a large mixed salad and 1 tbsp reduced-calorie dressing*

# INDEX

# ACKNOWLEDGEMENTS

This has been a special project for us and one we're very proud of. We'd like to say a big thank you to everyone who supported us through our diet and worked on the television series and this book.

Thanks to Lucie Stericker who pulled everything together creatively for the book and to Loulou Clark for doing a really fabulous job on the design. Thanks to our publisher Amanda Harris and our editor Jinny Johnson for helping us string our words together and encouraging us throughout. A big thank you to Lisa Harrison for all her skill in preparing the food for the photographs and to Andrew Hayes-Watkins for making it all look so lipsmackingly luscious – great job both of you. And a very special thank you to Justine Pattison for her inspirational help and advice on the recipes and for sharing her encyclopaedic knowledge of all things calorific – and not so calorific – with us. Thank you to our recipe-testing team, Gileng Salter, Lauren Brignell, Jane Gwillim, Fran Brown and Jane Rushworth for all your valuable feedback.

As always, thanks to all at James Grant Management for your continuing help and support on our projects.

Huge thanks to all the Optomen team who worked so hard on the television series: Alex, Eli, Dave, Susie, Kat, Laura and Nicola, our executive producer. Ian Denyer played the part of three men – director, producer and cameraman – and we'd like to thank him for his boundless energy and super-human efforts. Thanks to our gurus Professor Roy Taylor, aka Dr Doom, and Dr Ashley Adamson for inspiring us and not condemning us and for all your support and advice on weight loss. Thanks to the ever-cheerful Jane Gwillim, our home economist on the show, and to Sammy-Jo for putting in an appearance.

We'd also like to thank BBC commissioners Alison Kirkham and Lisa Edwards, and Janice Hadlow, controller of BBC Two, for going along with our ever-dafter ideas.

Last but not least, much love to all our Big Eaters who joined us on our journey, some more successfully than others. You know who you are!

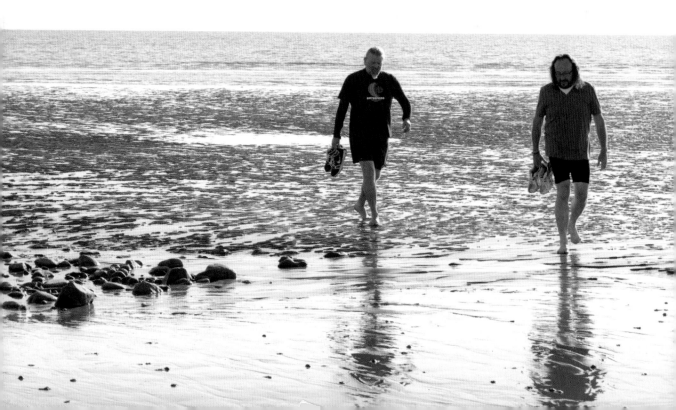